Creativity and Communication
in Persons with Dementia

For Sitar

Creativity and Communication in Persons with Dementia
A Practical Guide

With Much Love

John Killick and Claire Craig

John

Jessica Kingsley *Publishers*
London and Philadelphia

The image on the front cover is of stained glass and was designed by people with dementia as part of a project with occupational therapist Christine Davidson and her husband, a stained glass artist.

First published in 2012
by Jessica Kingsley Publishers
73 Collier Street
London N1 9BE, UK
and
400 Market Street, Suite 400
Philadelphia, PA 19106, USA

www.jkp.com

Library of Congress Cataloging in Publication Data
Killick, John, 1936-
  Creativity and communication in persons with dementia / John Killick and Claire Craig.
    p. ; cm.
  Includes bibliographical references and index.
  ISBN 978-1-84905-113-2 (alk. paper)
  1. Dementia--Treatment. 2. Art therapy. 3. Arts--Therapeutic use.
4. Interpersonal communication. I. Craig, Claire, 1969- II. Title.
  [DNLM: 1. Dementia--therapy. 2. Art Therapy--methods. 3. Communication.
4. Creativeness. 5. Dementia--psychology. WM 220]
  RC521.K5524 2011
  616.8'3--dc22
                                    2011010171

British Library Cataloguing in Publication Data
A CIP catalogue record for this book is available from the British Library

ISBN 978 1 84905 113 2
eISBN 978 0 85700 301 0

Printed and bound in Great Britain by Bell & Bain Ltd, Glasgow

For Kate, our friend who has been
an inspiration to both of us

Contents

Introduction

This book can be regarded as in some ways a sequel to *Communication and the Care of People with Dementia* written by John Killick with Kate Allan and published by Open University Press in 2001. That was a wide-ranging text, and our contribution, more modest in scale, concentrates on those aspects of communication related to creativity, which were touched on by that book but not explored in detail in its pages.

Another important parallel with that text is their exploratory nature. Both have been written in a spirit of enquiry rather than dogmatism. Although in the decade that has elapsed between the two volumes there have been advances in understanding of ways in which the arts can contribute to the lives of people with dementia, we still lack a body of evidence which can offer conclusive proof of that role. And though many projects, large and small, have been mounted in the intervening period, we believe we are still at the experimental stage in this area. Of course if anything like the money that has been poured into drugs research had come the way of the kinds of initiatives we describe, we might be in a very different situation today. But it is no good crying over spilt paint or lost chords; we hope to offer an honest account of the current state of play, and hope to inspire many to set out on the adventure in future.

We have designed the text in as helpful a way as possible. Part 1 raises fundamental questions and tries to offer some answers. The second, and longest part, introduces various art forms and suggests possibilities for employing them. Part 3 is an in-depth exploration of how to get things off the ground. The last part is a sequence of brief personal accounts of people and projects which we hope will help to keep the book focused. Some of the chapters were jointly composed, and some were the work of one or other of us, as is indicated by the names beneath the individual chapters. Each of the 14 chapters that make up Part 2 end with Try-outs, practical activities we hope will inspire you to do more than just reading.

We have given each of us a paragraph to introduce the other. Here is John's about Claire:

I have known Claire for 12 years, during which time she has risen in the ranks of Occupational Therapists to become a Senior Lecturer – well deserved, I think, for someone who has published six books, run many workshops, and inspired innumerable staff and family carers. She is one of the world's enthusiasts, bubbling over with ideas and humour, and it is a pleasure to be learning from her all the time.

Now for Claire's turn:

What can I say about John that hasn't already been said? During the 12 years I have known him I have heard people refer to him as 'artist' 'pioneer' 'sage' 'guru'(!). These superlatives may go some way to describing what he does and how he is regarded but they do not capture the essence of John: his generosity of spirit, sense of fun, his tireless energy and above all his dedication to giving voice to people with dementia. Setting out on any project with John is an adventure.

PART 1

Why the Arts?

1.

What is Creativity?

We must first define what we mean by 'creativity'. It is an umbrella term and can be applied to a variety of human concerns and in a variety of contexts. There is a sense in which any activity from cleaning a floor to flying an aeroplane can be regarded as creative if it is approached in an open-minded and experimental frame of mind. But here it is necessary to limit ourselves to specific subjects and ways of proceeding. Not all will necessarily apply to everything we discuss in this book, but a cluster of them will certainly be inherent in each topic and technique.

One component of the cluster is the idea of pursuing an activity for its own sake. Of course this can apply as much to ten-pin-bowling as collage-making, but it will be present throughout every chapter here.

As is the fact that there is a making process involved. Nothing was there at the beginning but at the end of the activity something, whatever its scope and quality, will have been achieved. What is more, a potential for creativity may have been realised. This in turn gives the opportunity for admiration and celebration. The occurrence of creativity is always to be welcomed, especially in people with dementia, where the possibilities for underachieving, for undermining, are endless and occurrences of it depressingly frequent.

One easily overlooked but incontrovertibly essential quality of every creative category that we consider, is that it must give pleasure. We are thinking here particularly of the participant, but the approbation of others may also occur. This is not to deny the reality of struggle with materials and concepts in the act of creation but such feelings should not predominate. A man who had made a poem with John said:

This is heaven, because for a lot of people it helps them. You do it as a one-to-one and that's right. I feel I'm very lucky because I've got something like poetry.

A woman who made a picture with Claire said:

We have been on a wonderful journey, you and I. What fun we've had, laughing and singing. Holding a rainbow in our hands.

Another vital characteristic is that it must be expressive. Many people with dementia need constant reassurance that their selfhood is intact, and the exploration of feeling-states is helpful to that process. At the same time, and somewhat paradoxically, concentration on an activity can lessen self-consciousness. It improves focus and excludes distraction.

The sense of time is suspended, and this emphasises the importance of the moment. A woman whom John observed in a day centre who chain-smoked completely forgot to ask for a cigarette throughout a one-hour art group, painting being an activity that commanded her absorption.

Lastly, and of special significance, and related to the last point, is the sense of flow which is often experienced. We consider this of such importance that we have given it a chapter on its own.

We are aware that creativity is often regarded as something only possessed by people of high intelligence and perhaps even genius, like a great mathematician or painter, and it is true that in his groundbreaking book *Creativity*, Mihaly Czikszentmihalyi (1996) builds up a picture of the concept based solely on nearly 100 interviews with outstanding talents in every field of human endeavour. But we wish to establish at the outset that it is a characteristic of the life of every one of us, and is capable of development to enhance our lives immeasurably. We should like to distinguish big C creativity, where individuals have devoted themselves to developing a specific talent to the highest degree possible (sometimes to the detriment of their wellbeing) to small c creativity, which is what we are exploring in this book, and which has the potential to enhance wellbeing, especially for those people with dementia who are chronically denied achievement and its consequent satisfactions in so many aspects of their lives.

It is worth pausing here for a moment to reflect on what has been said. The difficulty is that even the word 'creativity' carries with it all kinds of hidden assumptions and connotations which, if not addressed, can act as barriers to participation. Early experiences of the arts can be particularly formative with regard to our relationship with creativity and our perception of exactly what it means to be 'creative'. For instance, Betty Edwards (1993) in her book *Drawing on the Right Side of the Brain* writes:

> *Unthinking people sometimes make sarcastic or derogatory remarks about children's art. The thoughtless person may be a teacher, a parent, another child or perhaps an admired older brother or sister. Many adults have related to me their painfully clear memories of someone's ridiculing their attempts at drawing.* (Edwards 1993, pp.63–4)

The result is that even as you read this you will have an opinion as to what constitutes a creative act and whether or not you are a creative person. These views will in turn determine how you engage with creative media, your response towards your own work and to the work of others. It is therefore worth spending time exploring this, since the individuals you are working alongside may also at some time be wrestling with these questions. Claire has found it useful to imagine creativity as 'a thing', as a tangible object, and to step back, walk around it, view it from different angles, and ask searching questions about it. The following exercise can be a good place to start:

When you think about the word 'Creativity' what picture automatically pops up into your mind?

What would it sound like?

What would it taste like?

If it was a place, where would it be?

If it was a texture, how would it feel?

What would it smell of?

What if it was an item of clothing? How would you feel when you put it on?

If creativity could speak, what would it say? How would you respond?

Complete the following sentence:

Creativity is…

This final exercise is a good one to share both with people with dementia and with colleagues to gain a measure of their understanding of the term. When John, Claire and Kate Allan invited people at a summer school about creativity to respond to this sentence here are some of their answers:

Creativity is an open flower blossoming.

It is individuality within, open to others old and new.

It is a bowl of cherries of which you eat each one very slowly.

It is opening your mind to boundless possibilities.

It is your journey.

It is a stimulus to activate the stimulus of the mind and body.

It is a joy, a pleasure.

It is infectious – you will want more.

It is freedom which lets your heart sing.

It is a bird which soars in the air and lets your spirit fly.

There is much merit in this final approach since the problem with defining creativity too exactly is that in doing so it is possible to lose the essence of what it is. It is the equivalent of defining something as elusive and as all-encompassing as love. Words tend to fail us here and our definitions become too limiting, too restrictive. It is the equivalent of taking hold of a handful of sand: the tighter you squeeze, the more quickly it slips through your fingers.

Given our definitions of creativity, the question undoubtedly arises as to whether this is something that everyone possesses? We would argue that we all have an innate sense of creativity. You need only to think of the capacity of children for invention and imagination. Indeed, in the early years creative play is the medium through which we experiment, explore and learn about the world. As we grow older this creative play manifests itself in different ways: in our hobbies and pastimes, in the music we listen to, the literature we read, the poetry we write, the way we dress, in how we style our hair, the way we move, how we decorate our homes, even the way we sign our name. Creativity offers us a way to forge our identity, celebrate our uniqueness, and is one of the ways we can make our mark on the world.

Therefore we could also say that creativity involves bringing something of the inside out, a letting go. It is about personally putting something of our inner selves into the outer world, an idea that Anne Davis Basting (Basting and Killick 2003) encapsulates when she says:

To be creative is to draw on one's lived experiences and transform them into something new. (Basting and Killick 2003, p.8)

Creativity is an expression of who we are, and when the arts form the vehicle or the means of channelling this creativity, the end result can embody something of the artist and their facets of personality.

We end this chapter with three more quotations on the subject of creativity to set us all thinking:

Creativity represents a miraculous coming together of the uninhibited energy of the child with its apparent opposite and enemy: the sense of order imposed by the disciplined adult intelligence. (Norman Podhoretz)

There's always a clean slate, a fresh sheet of paper, a waiting space, a chance to have another shot at it tomorrow. (Herbert Block)

To exist is to change, to change is to mature, to mature is to go on creating oneself endlessly. (Henri Bergson)

2.

What the Arts Can Do

The novelist Jeanette Winterson (2010) has written:

Art in all its forms is an encounter with emotion – a big reason why we need art, not as a luxury and leisure activity, but as a daily balance to our fear of feeling, our fear of the consequences of feeling.

This may well be true for many of us. We live in a culture that values thought above feeling, with consequences which have created an imbalance in our psyches and a reluctance, even apprehension, when given the challenge of being creative.

With people living with dementia we may be faced with a rather different situation. Because intellectual capacity may have diminished, they may be thrown back on emotion, and so the arts can be a natural outlet for their reaction to all the experiences they are going through. There may also be less reluctance in giving a new expressive medium a try.

We shall consider a number of possible functions of art, concentrating on those which, we believe, have a special relevance to people with dementia. The first of these we can call internal dialogue. This may take the form of a kind of self-communing: the employment of an external medium for the purpose of what is essentially a private conversation. What is produced may not be intended or appropriate for sharing with others. It is giving shape and meaning to a complex of feelings which would otherwise remain unexamined. The result may be an improvement in functioning at a basic level and thus a greater containment and contentment.

A second function of art for people with dementia is that of outward communication. Many people seem locked inside themselves and the arts can provide a set of keys. We must not underestimate the importance of providing opportunities of this nature. Each artform has its own language, and many of these do not require words for their expressive functioning, and we have found that many people with dementia fall upon these languages with a new sense of purpose. They can be valuable for people to communicate with each other and with those without the condition. And the social potential of these activities is very great. Making a group poem or drama improvisation or collage brings people together with a common purpose, and there are many outstanding projects which are intergenerational and bring different age-groups together. We must have strategies for tackling isolation, and the arts can offer this in a variety of ways.

A third function of the arts for people with dementia, and this at a basic level, is to offer activity. Regrettably, for many people with the condition having something to do, having *anything* to do, is denied them. So an arts activity, with its elements of design and improvisation, even if it communicates little to others, becomes meaningful. By being creatively occupied one asserts one's right to an independent existence, and in however small a way exerts a degree of control over one's world.

The aesthetic is another aspect of art which is meaningful for people with dementia. To bring something beautiful into existence is a laudable aim, and if it is admired by others that is an added bonus. The value of the craft element of a making activity is not to be underestimated. As one lady put it in a poem she made with John:

> *People think that you*
> *need something beautiful*
> *to make a beautiful picture.*
> *But what you need is skill.*
> *And the eye to see*
> *that it is beautiful.*

This raises the question of whether, if people do not have the skill in the first place, they are capable of learning it. It is impossible to be dogmatic about this but we know of many examples of individuals with the condition mastering a technique and going on to exercise it at a high level.

Finally, arts activities may be thought of as psychologically therapeutic. Here we could be entering something of a minefield! At one end of the spectrum there is the formalised therapy offered by trained practitioners in specific artforms such as art, music or dance; these are planned interventions with recognised procedures and classified outcomes, used for assessment and diagnosis. At the other end is any opportunity for activity that can prove diverting and bring transitory relief; its effects are unlikely to be measured. The former professionals can be suspicious of the latter. What seems clear, however, is that most provision has the potential for increasing wellbeing.

Of course these five functions may all be operative at the same time, whether intended or not by those providing the opportunities. Claire gives an example of where the first and second functions clearly interact:

> *Sometimes individuals speak through the work to express their fears and worries. During a session using decoupage one lady, rejecting flowers and animals to adorn her box, chose instead a small girl dressed in Victorian costume. She placed the picture on the inside of the box and quickly closed the lid. Quite unprompted she told me, 'She feels very alone and frightened. What do you make of that?' I told her that it must be difficult, and she nodded her head slowly and said, 'Yes, I really miss my sister. I wish she could be here for me to talk to.'* (Craig 2001, p.36)

John was observing a puppetry group where one lady was obviously identifying with her puppet more closely than the other participants. Her enjoyment was palpable yet there was a serious content to her relationship with the character she was manipulating, which suddenly burst out in the following words, which John made into a poem:

He's not smart. It's the lady who put him there.
What kind of a person is he? I know:
He's a person who stands for something else.
This seems to be unique, the whole set-up of him.
Whereabouts was it born, do you know?

Thinking about a name? What is thought?
I think it is called Puppy Longwise
Because you don't know how long the wisdom's been there.
We're led to believe that he has no thought –
Do you have asservations like that?

And now I'm taking my hand away –
I want to see if he misses me.

No doubt an art therapist (or a poetry therapist) would be analysing this for what it tells them about the person's unconscious motivations, but we are content to consider it as a creative reflection on the process she has been experiencing. It probably partakes of aspects of all five of the functions we have identified. Certainly it explores excitingly the dual nature of a puppet (is it an object or a person?). Not least of the complexities here is that it represents the creation of one work of art in response to another artform.

Although this only applies to a small group of those with dementia, there is a very interesting piece of ongoing research by Professor Bruce Miller (2000) of the University of California. He discovered, almost by accident that there were some instances amongst those individuals with frontotemporal-lobe dementia of exceptional artistic talent, and that a handful of these people had never shown signs of such creativity before.

In the preface to his book of photographs James McKillop (2003) says this:

Being told I had dementia led to a door re-opening after a difficult time in my life. New challenges, new friendships. I wanted to raise awareness about dementia and show that people with dementia can re-learn forgotten skills as well as learn new ones.

The opportunity the arts provide to learn something new is frequently overlooked, partly because it is sometimes assumed that developing new skills or interests is somehow beyond the scope of people with dementia. We know this to be untrue. People with dementia have the capacity to learn new things or at the very least to engage in new opportunities, and we should not let our own preconceptions hinder this since the process can help to re-build self-esteem and offer the chance of the development of new roles. The arts have much to offer here, but we need to think carefully about how we support individuals to gain the most from these experiences. We go into some detail about this in Chapter 18.

There will be many people with dementia who are not aware of the possibilities that the arts provide for expressiveness and an increase in wellbeing. We need to develop careful strategies to introduce them to different artforms and what they offer. At the same time there are other individuals with the condition who are experiencing a marked sense of release, perhaps of disinhibition, and they may be already aware of what the arts could offer them. Agnes Houston, a woman with dementia in Scotland, reflects both of these characteristics:

> I'm not saying dementia's not serious. But I'm going to say that it's a licence in a way, a licence to be free, to be me. I think when I got the diagnosis I got permission to be more relaxed into this person and accept her.
>
> I wanted to find out if I was artistic. Creativity's an aspect I want to explore. Being able to feel out of the box is what I'm picking up. It will happen. It's a bit like waiting on Christmas. You know it's coming but as a child you don't know exactly when. It's a nice feeling. (Houston 2009)

There is one aspect of the therapeutic which we should not close this chapter without highlighting. It is one we can identify, but it will manifest itself in different ways in different individuals. We are referring to the way so many people with the condition find ways of coping with the various changes, some of them losses, which they experience. Anger, distress, denial – these are examples of how some people react. But we believe the arts can provide outlets for distressing feeling-states, which at the least can make circumstances more tolerable, and at their best can confer a whole new meaning on the processes being undergone. As Alida Gersie, an arts therapist and writer, says:

> *When we are engaged in symbolic expressive activities we do not have to accommodate ourselves to external demands or models; there are neither coercions nor sanctions and this enables the assimilation and therefore the transformation of experienced reality. When this reality is grievous it is of even greater importance that this process occurs.* (Gersie 1991, pp.235–236)

3.

Getting in the Flow

What does the concept of 'flow' mean to you? The word can be used in a variety of contexts. It is what a river does, constant and unstoppable. We speak of the movement of a dress as 'flowing', meaning the whole of the garment moves as one, all the parts contributing to the whole. We speak of being 'in the flow', which presupposes there is a place where it is all happening, and where we want to be. In common with all these is the idea of a central experience in which everything hangs together.

When did you last experience anything of this kind? What did it feel like? Was there a sense of achievement at the end of it?

Anyone who has brought up children knows how aggravating it can seem when they are told to be ready for an outing or a meal, but when the time comes they are so absorbed in an activity that they have failed to make any preparation. Children have fewer responsibilities than adults so they find it easier to practise a concentration dependent upon the blanking out of other aspects of the environment or of the awareness of personal identity. But we all have heightened experiences of this kind, and perhaps could have more if we valued them more and gave ourselves, or were presented with, more opportunities to enjoy them. Unfortunately in western society greater emphasis is placed on logical processes than those where the different aspects of consciousness are integrated. There seems to be an inherent suspicion of a concept like flow as perhaps possessing mystical attributes.

The psychologist Mihaly Czikszentmihalyi (pronounced cheek-sent-me-high) has spent most of his career trying to answer questions about flow and gathering data to identify common factors. Amongst those he has verified are the following:

1. A certain level of skills is in operation.

2. The degree of challenge offered is commensurate with one's level of ability.

3. There is instant feedback on performance.

4. The activity is judged as worthwhile in itself – although there may be awareness of an outcome it is not considered the be-all-and-end-all.

5. There is a sense of being in total control – that whatever challenges the activity throws up, one will be able to cope.

6. The degree of concentration exercised is such that awareness of events outside the task are very much lessened, and one's consciousness of self almost erased.

7. The sensation of time passing is temporarily suspended. (Czikszentmihalyi 2008)

A distinction needs to be made between flow and pleasure. We all need pleasure in our lives, and whether it is obtained through eating or sleeping or sex it has a restorative quality: an imbalance or lack has been remedied. But pleasure does not of itself promote growth. Flow is a much more complex phenomenon than pleasure. Flow has many dimensions: thoughts, intentions, actions and the senses all contribute to the experience, and in their coming together something new and richer is created. A new order in the psyche is established: flow experiences make a contribution to maturity.

A phrase used by Nakamura and Czikszentmihalyi is that of being in 'dynamic equilibrium'. Research has shown that interaction between the person and their environment is an important factor in the experience, and this results in a state where the person responds to what happened immediately before in the process rather than any pre-existing drive or plan. It is a matter of subjectively perceived opportunities. Performance is regulated by inner resources discovered at the time rather than any remembered capacities; this is a characteristic of particular significance where people with dementia are concerned. The experience of flow is one of integration, whereas it appears that in many instances the experience of dementia is one of disintegration – the different aspects of the person failing to add up to a coherent whole. Flow gives the person with the condition the opportunity, however temporary, to feel together again. It is inherently pleasurable and promotes growth. Nakamura and Czikszentmihalyi also stress the health-giving aspects of flow and the enhancement of self-esteem. They end their article with the sentence:

> *Although it seems clear that flow serves as a buffer against adversity and prevents pathology, its major contribution to the quality of life consists in endowing momentary experience with value.* (Nakamura and Czikszentmihalyi 2005, p.102)

Since by force of circumstance people with dementia are obliged to live largely in the moment, it is difficult to exaggerate the importance of this concept in the development of strategies for helping them to live fulfilling lives.

The sixth characteristic listed above is also of special significance where people with dementia are concerned. If it is accepted that the sense of self is threatened by dementia, then experiences where that sense and its threat are subsumed into something more absorbing may bring relief from conflict and loss if only temporarily. But it is claimed that flow can do more for the person than straightforward distraction. Czikszentmihalyi (2008) claims that what is involved is the possibility for self-transcendence. So what may come back after the activity is over is different from what was there before: a sense of self-enhancement, and this flow carries within it the seeds of strengthening the self for persons with the condition. It would be good to have confirmation of this process through research, but unfortunately it has not yet been done. But we cannot wait for this to happen: there is sufficient evidence from common observation for us to proceed. Enough that there appears to be a psychological mechanism at work here: we should concentrate on finding the right experiences of flow for each individual.

A woman John worked with many times in a nursing home producing poems asked him one day, *'Would you please give me back my personality?'* It shocked him because he only had experience of her in the context of deep conversations when she was clearly functioning at her optimum level, in other words, demonstrating flow. At other times, however, she must have been struggling with changes in the way she thought and felt, and these were reflected in other exclamations such as, *'It's the terrific confusion of things that worries me more than anything else'* and, *'The brilliance of my brain has slipped away when I wasn't looking.'* The process of talking released these insights, but it also encompassed more positive evaluations of her situation like, *'People try so hard to get us in a normal situation. It comes over me in a distinct feeling of joy.'* It seems to us that getting people in a normal situation is a special contribution that flow can make to the lives of people with dementia.

A fascinating article by Lesley Benham (2008) tells how a dull corner of a nursing home was transformed, with the assistance of the residents, into a stimulating display area. She comments on two women with dementia combining forces on carrying out a particular creative task:

> *Neither required much guidance as they became absorbed in the challenge. They were totally occupied with the task, showing increased concentration and improved communication skills throughout the sessions. Noticeably, word-finding and fluency seemed to improve as they were under no direct pressure to converse or give opinions. Conversation was spontaneous and humour flowed.*
> (Benham 2008, p.16)

A man working on his own on the same kind of task (in his case he was painting a wall) displayed similar absorption:

> *Engrossed in the task, he worked under minimal direction for days, recoating the area. Watching him, no-one would have believed this man experienced memory problems and other health issues — he was so energetically and proudly engaged in constructive work.* (Benham 2008, p.16)

Clearly, the arts is an area where people with dementia can be presented with creative activities that fulfil all the criteria for flow. We can only imagine what a world full of challenges carefully selected to suit the person would be like. It could well constitute a transformation scene. We wonder if this was what the lady in the 'Memories in the Making' project was experiencing when, after a session of watercolour painting, she said, *'I don't know why so many things I always did are so hard now and THIS is so easy.'* (Jenny and Oropeza 1993, p.93)

PART 2
What's on Offer?

4.

The Food of Love
The Language of Music

John Killick

'Darling, they're playing our tune' – this familiar cry is redolent of melodies, voices and performances towards which couples have developed a sentimental attachment. When one of the partners is no longer there the music often retains the capacity to occasion a smile or a tear. This is the most basic level of adult musical response, and not to be undervalued. We must give people the opportunity to hear, respond to, and sing what is most familiar. We shall return to singing later in the chapter.

If nostalgia was all that music had to offer people with dementia their lives would be impoverished indeed. Let us set against the scenario above the following account. It comes from a transcript of a session run by Maria Mullan, a musician working in care homes and day centres in Northern Ireland. She and a participant have just been duetting on a glockenspiel. She then plays a solo piece:

Bob: *You touch the very, the little strings as I think in the centre of my heart. What do you think of that now?*

Maria: *I touch the strings in the centre of your heart? Is that how you feel when you listen to the music?*

Bob: *Oh yes, Oh yes I do, yes. There's something in you, like, I suppose mental as well naturally and I don't know, you can't explain it, that's the way it is.*

Bob's reaction reminds us how important it is to find the right piece of music for the person. Too often, particularly in residential settings, little care is taken to consider the tastes of individuals.

Playing music together has a special role in providing individuals with creative opportunities. In an article Mullan (2005) quotes another participant as follows:

> *Playing this instrument it really responds to me. I feel I fit in so beautifully. I feel I'm being drawn into another world. It's not just playing, there's part of yourself in that.* (Mullan 2005)

Mullan is not a music therapist, though her approach has something in common with the professional practice of therapists in the way she gives the person their head to improvise in their own way. But there's no element of the diagnostic in her method. (If you are interested in the music therapy approach we can recommend an article by Powell and O'Keeffe – see References.)

We must stress here, as elsewhere, that it is unnecessary to be a trained musician, let alone a therapist, to initiate valuable musical experiences with people with dementia, though as in any arts activity some experience helps.

For individuals with more serious communication difficulties music can still fulfil a positive function in their lives, though they may be unable to play even the simplest percussion instrument. It may well require a more proactive approach on the part of the initiator, but the rewards can be remarkable. Lois McCloskey (1990) is a musician in America who first researches a person's past life and then builds the session round it:

> *One way of affirming the quality of a person's life is to acknowledge that person's gifts and experiences. I validate them through music. I sing to them about their lives. I sing about the people they have*

touched, those they have loved, and contributions they have made throughout their lives. I sing so that they may begin to let go and release themselves from pain. (McCloskey 1990)

The above is an example of singing to the person by a musician. What are the effects on them by a caregiver? In a research project in Sweden (Brown *et al.* 2001) professional staff sang popular and folk songs to individuals in a dementia unit whilst carrying out basic tasks. The results were notable, and some of the benefits they identified were as follows:

1. It was a simple but effective method.

2. There was little or no cost involved.

3. It was a natural expansion of the caregiver role.

4. It was applicable in any kind of care setting.

5. It could be used by any kind of caregiver.

6. It could be adapted to suit the individual.

7. It resulted in markedly increased cooperation by the person being cared for.

8. It significantly enhanced the caregiving relationship.

9. It improved the caregiver's motivation and reduced burnout.

10. It could be co-ordinated with any music therapy programme. (Brown *et al.* 2001)

Singing by the person with the condition can be especially important. One day I was visiting a nursing home and had been told that Ella loved singing. She had worked as a vocalist in clubs in her younger days, and still had a fine, strong voice. I made contact with her, and at my request she began to sing. The melody was a familiar one, and the voice quality and projection were intact, but the words were unrecognisable. She reminded me of a Scottish folksinger improvising Gaelic as in 'mouth-music'. My rough transcript read:

> *Ay to the boy to the way to the way*
> *At the way to the way at doder doder may*
> *At the doder little ohti doder day*
> *At the old wey hey the idle didle day*
> *At the older dodle day.*

I had recorded her, and I played the recording back to her. To my surprise she sang along to the tape, reproducing the exact sounds she had made the first time. Although the words made no sense to me they clearly did to Ella. I provide this anecdote in order to stress that we have to find what process suits the person, however unconventional it may seem.

In recent years the formation of choirs for people with dementia has grown apace. Many of these exist under the umbrella term for the movement 'Singing For the Brain' (started by Chreanne Montgomery-Smith 2006). Obviously the organisation of such an initiative requires a good deal of planning. The venue must be suitable, and the leader carefully chosen. People with dementia and their carers are invited.

Amongst the characteristics of such choirs are:

1. Sessions begin with a warm-up routine.

2. Concentration and attention are challenged through complex working with songs.

3. The emotional content of songs is emphasised to make them more memorable.

4. Participants' confidence in most instances grows apace.

5. Relationships between people with dementia and their carers are enhanced.

6. Individuals are empowered by taking on roles.

7. Stress is reduced.

Turtle Key Arts is a company in London that collaborates with other organisations to mount innovative projects. They have been working in association with English Touring Opera and the Royal College of Music in a series of events called 'Turtle Song'.

A group of people with dementia and their carers meet once a week for a limited period to sing together, compose a song cycle, and record a CD. Examples of the imaginative outcomes can be seen on their website: www.turtlekeyarts.org.uk under 'education and participation'.

In their article on music therapy Powell and O'Keeffe (2010) describe vividly the therapeutic benefits of group work, and their comments are equally applicable to choirs set up for people with dementia outside that framework:

> *In music therapy groups the music welcomes and warms, encouraging interaction and listening, and encompassing different needs – comforting, relaxing, enlivening, surprising. A visitor to a session once described a music therapy group as me (the therapist) 'picking up threads' (participants' initiations) and weaving them together. This seems an apt description – weaving a piece of music. The 'warp and weft' of the musical 'cloth' connects and holds people together. I remember a woman with dementia who had just finished a song, once asking the group, 'Shall I knit you another one?' Doesn't this express how it might feel to have the fragments of thought or experience brought together in music?*

To sum up, I cannot do better than quote a number of people with dementia in conversation with John:

> *That song, it may be partial*
> *but you can tell it's nice.*
> *I like it so long as it doesn't*
> *leave off and forget the actual.*
> *When I'm with someone singing like this,*
> *you know, it always fills me up.*

★

> *I used to sing for the people,*
> *sing what fits the emotion at the time.*
> *When I first did it*
> *I thought I was going to be reprimanded*
> *for singing out of line.*
> *But Life is Singing.*

You can build it up as you go,
you can stand up and sing with it –
it's a question of feeling, of hearing, of saying YES!

TRY-OUTS

Listen to a range of music. As you do so, imagine what the composer was trying to say/convey when he wrote this. See if you can find another piece of music that could respond to this.

Now find a piece of music that somehow expresses how you feel at this precise moment.

Imagine you are on the radio programme Desert Island Discs – what four pieces of music would you choose and why?

What piece of music would be your signature tune?

5.

Moving in the Moment

Dance

John Killick

In the previous chapter we saw how music and dance are closely allied. A feeling induced by a piece of music can easily and effortlessly be translated into movement. Maybe it is a rhythm that causes the limbs to move; maybe it is a memory of an event that causes the body to sway. Farleigh defines dance as, *'an aesthetic (affectively vital) expression of the lived body; it is life engendering.'* Penny Greenland (2009), the founder of JABADAO, the earliest provider of dance training for those working with people with dementia in the UK, puts it this way:

> *Dancing is an ordinary and fundamental human activity hidden by a culture that has little regard for spontaneous movement as an expression of who we are and how we feel, in favour of more intellectual means. By dancing I don't mean steps and forms – I mean the spontaneous movements that ripple out of us all, sometimes consciously and sometimes unconsciously. They are our body's response to everything we do and see: movement waiting to be formed and shared if we choose to do so.* (Greenland 2009)

Richard Coaten (2007), one of the most thoughtful and innovative of a younger generation of dance therapists, stresses the body's memory bank in his account of the subject:

> *What makes dance and movement so important is that its expression is close to the source and location of all those buried memories – in the skin, cells, muscles and tissues of the body as much as the parts of the brain where this information gets stored. For people with cognitive impairment and difficulties in communication verbally, the opportunities offered by a different, non-verbal way of communicating may be of great importance.* (Coaten 2007, pp.19–22)

Can only dance therapists give individuals and groups this fundamental experience? Heather Hill, a dance therapist in Australia, thinks not. In her essential text *Invitation to the Dance* (Hill 2001) she expresses her belief that it is not necessary to have extensive dance training, although you do need responsiveness to music and a certain lack of inhibition with regard to movement. She does not see inexperience as any great barrier, but you should be willing to learn. Your own dancing ability can be modest but you need to be of a playful nature. You must possess the attributes of flexibility and positivity. She takes us through the practicalities of running a session, including length, the size of a group and the venue. She places particular emphasis on the space in which the activity is to occur: it must be of an adequate size and welcoming, and above all every participant must be able to find their own space within it. She enumerates the various aspects of the session: the greetings, the warm-up, the pacing, the theme, and the winding-down. She emphasises trust, inclusiveness and relationship.

There is a section full of vivid portraits of individuals gaining benefit from the activity, here is one of them:

> *Mr J, in the four years he spent at the nursing home, was always one of the hardest of the residents to make contact with – except in the dance. While usually closed within himself, except in those moments when suspicion and distrust of staff actions would make him lash out, he seemed to open up in the dance sessions. He would watch,*

smile and then even get up to dance. The unit manager commented that Mr J 'lived for the dance sessions.' Time and dementia, however, took their toll and eventually Mr J became quite immobilised and even further shut away in himself. He would spend the day lying in a big armchair in rigid immobility staring into space or sleeping. However, he would still come to dance and often, but not always, he might have eye contact or raise a hand to hit the ball or take a staff member's hand. One day I felt moved to sing to him Brahms' Lullaby in German, not his native language. It is probably a sentimental favourite of many Europeans. As I sang, he began to cry – I just held him and gently rocked with him. When we returned to the ward his wife was there and Mr J said something to her in his native language. It was only later that I learned he had told his wife, 'I've been dancing with tears in my eyes.' (Hill 2001)

In an article memorably titled *A Space to Be Myself* Hill (2003) provides the following quotes from Elsie, one member of a group of whom she made a special study:

Thank you for bringing me out of my shell.

I've got together again.

It's brought the dullness out of me… to the brightness.

And I think it's brought me out of… Wake up.

So that's brought me out of my cupboard. (Hill 2003, p.39)

In an article specifically concentrating on the link between dance and memory, Richard Coaten (2007) describes the response of Mabel, an attendee at a day centre, to a session involving music and movement and objects:

We introduced ourselves and began a gentle physical warm-up, rubbing hands together, tapping our feet and moving gently to the music. The theme for the morning was 'Washday' and before long we passed round an object to help focus minds and memories. Mabel took the carpet-beater in her hands and there was an expectant silence. She drew it up close between her fingers, feeling the warmth of the wood and the familiarity of the shape.

She turned it over and over, rocking a little as her memory stirred. Here was a small, quiet dance full of past life, present pleasure and the experience of beauty. The others watched. It was touching and beautiful to see.

Mabel's mood changed. She shared the fragment of a memory about being chased playfully around the back-court by her father when she was a girl. A laugh sprang out of that story, followed by another and another. The beauty of the object and the still, quiet dance had given Mabel back a sense of herself. She left the room feeling very different and told staff how much she had enjoyed the session. (Coaten 2007)

Later in his article Coaten comments:

The process appears not to be about re-enacting a past event or memory so much as re-living it in the present. The living symbol of the original event manifests in the moment. (Coaten 2007)

The kind of dance we have been describing so far could be called 'pure expressive movement'. Much more familiar to most people is social dance in its various forms, and of these the most popular with the older generation is ballroom dancing. There are people close to their diagnosis of dementia who are still able to participate in such sessions, and it is particularly valuable for couples. Oliver Sacks in his chapter on dementia in his book *Musicophilia* comments:

When we dance together bonding is deeper. Moving together helps to regain a sense of physical identity. (Sacks 2007)

Where individuals are no longer mobile they can be encouraged to move to the music in their chairs or wheelchairs.

In 1999 Dorothy Jerrome published an article outlining the benefits of the first Circle Dance sessions she had run, and this is a movement that has quickly spread. Many groups now exist, and there are training courses for staff. The dances are an invention based on folkdances from a variety of countries. Russia, Greece, South America, the Balkans, Israel and Celtic countries have all been drawn upon, but the movements and rhythms have been simplified for ease of learning and performance. Recorded music is used, and it has its own stimulating and healing properties. The measured processing and holding and rocking have something of the quality of ancient ritual. The togetherness engendered is profoundly supportive and reassuring to the participants, and can also benefit relatives and staff. As Jerrome (1999) says:

> One of the most humbling experiences of dancing with people with dementia is a sense of shared vulnerability. When dancing we also occasionally experience being flooded with feeling – overwhelming sadness or anger or euphoria – apparently 'out of the blue'. Such feelings come from the experiential self, reached directly by the music and dance. This puts us, briefly and valuably, on the same emotional plane as the people we look after. (Jerrome 1999)

TRY-OUTS

As you walk and sit start to pay attention to how you move; the length of your stride, your pace, the swing of your arm. Try varying this in some way. For instance, lengthening your stride or pausing momentarily before you sit down. Register how that makes you feel. You could add to this, so that the way you walk or sit becomes part of your own movement signature.

Our hands are incredibly expressive. Try having a conversation with someone using only your hands, no speech. How does this make you feel?

We hear it described that people 'jump for joy'. Can you express how you feel by moving in a certain way? See if other people can identify the emotion.

6.

Giving Voice
Writing Poetry

John Killick

You are words. Words can make or break you. Sometimes people don't listen, they give you words back, and they're all broken, patched up. But will you permit me to say that you have the stillness of silence, that listens, and lasts.

★

You say what you've got in your heart, and that's enough.

★

I find it absolutely overwhelming that I've got all this bubbling up inside and then someone comes along who actually wants me to give him all the specific details of what Alzheimer's like, rather than having their eyes glazed over when I rabbit on about myself all the time.

These are statements by persons with dementia about the significance of poetry writing for them.

In only a very few instances are people actually able to write the poem down for themselves – I must do the writing for them. But that makes the process an even more significant one, in my view, for people otherwise tend to be locked in their own minds and sensibilities, and my presence is giving them a voice. As one member of staff in a care home put it, having observed my role: *'You are a linguist of lost words.'* What follows is a brief description of how I go about this work.

The process involves first of all making a relationship with the person: this often takes only a few minutes. I try to get on their wavelength, I make it clear I am there for them, and they can talk about anything that interests them. At a certain point, when intimacy and fluency have been achieved, I may ask permission to write down or tape-record their words. Occasionally a poem is achieved then and there. Usually it is a matter of taking away their words and working on them. There is one important exception however, (and this is the first golden rule): I add nothing, only take away. I am looking for the emotional thread in their discourse and hoping to make it clear, whilst only employing the language they have used.

It is important not to force the poem into a straitjacket provided by rhyme and metre. These are prose utterances with a poetic quality, and it is important to preserve speech rhythms wherever possible. You will need to make decisions about line-endings and dividing up the text into verses. The poetic quality I refer to is often contributed to by metaphor. The American poet Sharon Olds (2009) says, *'I don't have an imagination. I have an "image-ination", in that images come through me into my poems.'* I think some people with dementia operate in this way, as the poems quoted below will illustrate.

I take back the poem and share it with the person. They are given a copy and I read it to them. I ask their opinion of it, and their permission to share it with others (friends and relatives, care staff, a wider audience). If permission is granted for any level of sharing a form is signed for release of the poem. I keep the copyright on behalf of the person, or it may be held by the organisation for which I am working.

As can be imagined, reactions to the poem may vary. At one extreme there can be a rejection of the poem as worthless or a denial of its authorship. At the other extreme comes the injunction

'Publish it!' The second golden rule is to abide by the person's decision. Sometimes relatives step in and make the decision on behalf of the person.

The majority of people appear to value the process tremendously. It is a confirmation for them that their words are being taken seriously, and a confirmation for readers that it is worth communicating with people with dementia.

So what are the poems that I am presented with (and which I re-present to the person) like? It is time I gave some examples. I will set each one in its context. The first is short and seemingly straightforward in its message, but I will suggest that it is more complex and profound than it may appear. The scene is a care home lounge. A man is sitting alone; he is looking around agitatedly; he voices his fears to me:

The Key

Have you any openings?
Have you got a guide?
Could you come along
and turn a key in a lock for me?

You'll not find my room.
I've only got nothing.

This my room? Not mine.
Not my room.
Not my clothes.
Not my bed.

I'm going home.

This is emotion reduced to its essence. Every word is the man's. I don't believe he is asking for a real key, as we are nowhere near any doors. In any case, you would not normally use expressions like 'openings' or 'a guide' to ask someone to open a door. I suggest that this is symbolic language and not to be interpreted literally. Under the force of feeling this man is using metaphor to embody his distress. If we examine the final line, this cannot be interpreted in a straightforward manner either. He makes no attempt to leave. Perhaps he is expressing a wish to be in his own home rather than the institution in which he finds himself? Or is this a more profound expression of unease at his mental condition, a cry from the heart that his world is broken and he wants it mended?

Here is another poem, by a woman this time; she is looking out of the window of the care home at the world outside:

Freedom

Are we all kidnapped?
I'm not at all sure
what kidnapping is, but
I know I'm very frightened.

I could go out there
and sit on that swing
and I would enjoy it.
I want my freedom.

But we none of us have our freedom.
I don't understand so much
that I'll just do without it,
chuck the whole lot in the air.

In some ways this poem is even simpler than 'The Key' – a plea for understanding the process she is going through. But there is still room for metaphor: the idea of kidnapping is a potent one, and though sitting on the swing would be a practical act, it also represents a whole host of possibilities which may have been denied the person by the condition or the way people treat the person with the condition.

I think the main reason that poetry writing is so important for many people with dementia is that the condition has a disinhibiting effect. At the same time that intellectual capacities are diminished and rational language proves elusive, suddenly talk blooms with allusion; the currents of feeling are reflected in rhythm and cadence. I believe that for the individual poetry writing provides release and an opportunity to come to terms with a process that can seem overwhelming, a ravelling that demands to be unravelled. Here is a poem by a man on this very subject:

Using my Brain

What I've done this year is a thinking process.
I'm now coming back to the land of questioning things.

It's important you think the right things
or you turn in upon yourself.

This is the phase when I need to be opening outwards.

Some of the poems express a yearning sense of the spiritual. A man in a nursing home lounge one day asked if I had my notebook with me and dictated the following:

In the skies up high
with the clouds below you –
that's where I'd like to be.

With the birds,
the little sparrows,
but I'll remain a man.

It's an attraction,
it's the spaces
that we can't reach.

I was up there one day
and got the sensation
I didn't want to come down.

I'd rather be
a creature of the air
than of the earth.

When I asked him if he had a title he said, 'The Blue Far Yonder' in a tone of voice that suggested it was something I should have known!

Kerry Mills is a manager for the Hearthstone Foundation in America (see Chapter 17) and describes how she uses poetry to enhance awareness of communication in training sessions for staff.

The passages below are quoted from private correspondence, with her permission.

I have been working with about 50 nursing home staff including nurses, certified nursing assistants and housekeepers. The last exercise we do is to talk about listening. I point out how rewarding it is when there is someone who will listen to us. Then I tell them about you and I read them the poem you edited called 'My Dream'.

After I give everyone a paper and a pencil I ask them to go and sit with one resident. I ask them not to ask specific questions like how many children do you have and where are you from, but rather how are you today or how do you feel or what are you thinking? And then listen to what the resident has to say. Well the whole thing created a response in staff that I hadn't expected. My goal was that they would understand why people with dementia act the way that they do and that so much of their behaviour is simply because they are people. For some this was the case. But for some, they ended up seeing themselves as the same. For these people it was the listening exercise that allowed them to make this connection. One young CNA man (probably 23 years old) came back and said that he too writes poetry. He handed me the poem he had made from the words of the resident, and said that he himself could have written it:

> *Sometimes I don't know what I'm doing*
> *Sometimes I feel kind of bad*
> *I wish I knew*
> *Thanksgiving Day my legs got twisted on the side*
> *A truck hit me*
> *It started hurting*
> *I don't know what to say*
> *I'll tell you the truth*
> *I know one thing, I just feel bad*
> *I am hurting all over*
> *I feel better today though than yesterday.*

The young man said that this is how HE often feels. Another person, a nurse with a hard shell, came back and said that after she talked with her lady, she hugged her. She said she got as much out of the hug as the lady did and began to cry. The method of sitting and listening is so needed and so neglected in care. But it is so humanising.

Note: The poems come from John's books, as listed in the References.

TRY-OUTS

Sit with someone with dementia, and let them talk for at least 15 minutes. Ask if you may write down some of what they say, then read it back to them. Can you make a poem out of any of this?

Find an anthology of modern poems (*Staying Alive* edited by Neil Astley and published by Bloodaxe Books would be a useful choice) and find a poem that expresses something that you feel. Now shut the book and write your own feelings in poetic form.

7.

Making It All Up

Improvisation and Other Dramas

John Killick

Although it is possible in certain circumstances for people with dementia to perform scripted plays or to take part in play-reading, the challenges these activities pose for most people are so severe that, with limited space at our disposal, we have decided to devote the whole of this chapter to forms of improvisation.

'Making it all up' could have been invented for people with dementia. It is all in the moment, and this plays to their strengths. It is exciting, lively, frequently hilarious, and appears to have the effect of relaxing people and encouraging close relationships between the participants. I have organised a series of workshops of this kind in five different centres in Scotland (Killick 2003), for people who had been recently diagnosed, and here I provide a blow-by-blow account of what occurred.

I had taught improvised drama before in a college, so I drew on that experience. I also read texts by the great Brazilian Augusto Boal (1979, 1992, 1995), who had worked with the oppressed in his native country. And I made things up in the spirit of spontaneity that prevailed. I wanted to concentrate on humour as a way of breaking down barriers between people, so I called them 'Funshops'.

I decided to run a drama class in the first part of each three-hour session tailored to the participants, and this was a very active time involving everyone. Amongst the activities that proved most successful were:

walking around greeting each other

in pairs making each other laugh without using words

mirroring

creating statues (solo and group)

Grandmother's Footsteps (a form of group hide-and-seek)

object identification with eyes closed

talking gibberish

smelling a flower

miming professional occupations and

Accusation and Defence (where one partner accused the other of some misdemeanour, and the other had to justify his behaviour).

Then we would have a meal, a communal occasion which released many stories. We used these in the second half of the session, sometimes featuring the storyteller and sometimes directed by him/her. Although I had expected to play the role of observer at this juncture it was frequently demanded that I play a part. At every stage of the proceedings I encouraged humour to be used, and this lessened self-consciousness and increased enjoyment.

One man who had come apologising for his lack of a sense of humour, at the close complained that his sides hurt with laughing. Among comments have been the following:

I wouldn't miss this for the world. It has such a friendly atmosphere. Nobody singles you out. We're all in it together.

It's not just being silly. It's being serious. There's something serious behind this. When I sit on my own at night I think about it. I think about what has been said. And it helps.

One of the byproducts of 'The Funshops' has been 'The Chatshow'; it is a stand-alone activity that can assume an extended form. One person is chosen as host, and then has the task of choosing who is to be interviewed and on what aspects of their life. This can either be played straight or treated as a send-up of the TV format. Taken seriously, everyone learns a great deal about each other (including staff about their clients) in a short space of time. The rest of the group act as audience and laugh and clap in the appropriate places. (I should add that clapping is encouraged throughout the Funshop at every possible juncture, as a celebration of people's talents and personalities.)

Julie Kerton, a staff nurse in a day centre who has tried out the Chatshow idea comments:

I was absolutely amazed at how well it went. The interviewer and the interviewee got into role really easily and quickly forgot that we were watching. We felt really privileged to be listening to them. The great thing was, the activity has had lasting effects, as these two people have found things in common and begun to form a new friendship. (Kerton, private correspondence)

In one of the Funshops a greater interest was shown in scripted work. Sketches were tried out, but the monologue form held most appeal. Five monologues were produced, four written by myself in consultation with the individuals, and a fifth by the participant herself. They were then performed and filmed.

Also using humour most effectively in helping to draw people out is the Elderflowers Project, also run in Scotland. This employs trained actors, gives them knowledge of communication with people with dementia, and sends them into hospitals to help enliven people on the wards. The approach is not to perform at people but to draw them out, to help them to exercise their own senses of humour. In the following description Ian and Maria are the actors; Bob, Sandy, Kate and Emma live on the ward:

Bob reveals he was a naval man. Ian immediately volunteers for service. *'Would they take me?'* he asks. Bob looks him up and down. *'Ah well'*, he sighs *'anything's better than nothing.'* Ian has to learn saluting, but Bob declines to teach him. *'I don't do that'*, he explains, *'I get them to do it for me.'* Ian tries to teach himself, but in true clown tradition keeps falling over or hitting himself in the eye.

Maria volunteers and is also accepted as a trainee. This doubles the opportunity for incompetence in marching and saluting. Bob comments drily to the rest of the group, *'They'd be ideal to be on duty on Monday.'* However silly their antics, he never gets cross with them – he is playing along.

'Now, scrub the decks!' he orders. Ian and Maria do so vigorously. When they get up they rub their sore knees. Everyone is encouraged to rub their knees. Then to rub other people's knees. *'Oo, you nearly broke my fancy!'* jokes Sandy.

After the deck-scrubbing, Ian and Maria have to climb a mountain to improve their fitness. They mime the whole process. *'Not good enough'*, roars Bob, *'Now you have to climb a higher one!'* He points to an imaginary peak in the hospital grounds. *'If I join up today can I be an admiral tomorrow?'* asks Ian. Wearily, Bob can see no objection.

After their exertions Ian and Maria are very thirsty. In the corner of the room lie some skittles. *'Milk bottles over there – drink from them,'* shouts Kate. Ian and Maria swig gratefully.

As she leaves at the end of the session Emma says, *'They're a lot of fun. You can look around, and you don't need to go out for it, it's all in here.'*

'Elderflowers' provides one kind of interactive theatre; 'Ladder to the Moon' another. We have included a picture of Ladder to the Moon in the colour section. This is a London-based theatre company which functions in care settings. We almost wrote 'performs' because there is more of an element of 'the show' in their interventions. Although they too usually involve two actors, there is a story, usually taken from a Shakespeare play or a classic film, but around this dialogue an action is improvised. Sue Benson describes the process by which the people with dementia are involved in the action:

> *This is what makes their work distinct – active but sensitive seeking out of those who may seem to be less engaged and drawing them in. The way residents are invited to play roles is crucial. They are not explicitly asked if they would like to play the character, but approached and addressed in role – for example, 'My lord' or 'my gracious queen', with a bow and the offer of a crown – and the reaction tells the actor whether or not the role is accepted. The person is usually delighted, if bemused at first, and visibly grows in stature.* (Benson 2009)

Actor Susan Harvey described how the actors have become braver with experience of working with people with dementia. Where their instinct might have been to pick more alert, lively people to play leading roles, choosing those who seem less outgoing (at first sight) has brought great rewards. After a performance of 'A Very Greek Romance' (an adaptation of Troilus and Cressida) an activity co-ordinator observed: *'The lady who played the Queen is deteriorating daily; and today we saw a different person: she was attentive, involved and appropriate; she came in on cue, she exceeded everyone's expectations of her.'* (Harvey 2009, p.20)

It may be objected that both the previous examples depended upon the skills of professionals and their level of expertise is beyond that of most family carers and staff. This is true, but there is an openness and daring we can learn from them, and if you stop to analyse some of your own interactions with individuals and groups of people with dementia you may be surprised how many elements of playfulness and role playing you will find. A greater consciousness of the possibilities in this area can bear fruit in many situations.

To conclude, in a day centre I once saw a man, and a very upright character indeed in daily life, assume the role very convincingly of a two-timer. But he must have surprised himself, because he was at pains afterwards to assure his companions that he was really clean-living. We can only speculate at the psychological power involved in, if only for a few minutes, donning the mantle of another.

TRY-OUTS

The hidden life of an object. Choose an object. Spend time gaining a sense of its weight, texture, the material it is made of. How did this object come to be in your possession? If this object could speak, what would it say? How would it sound? Now imagine that it wants to become something else? What would that something else be?

If you could be a character in a play who would that character be and why?

If someone made your life into a play what type of play would it be? Would it be a comedy, a romance, a tragedy? Which actor/actress would you ask to play your part?

Go clothes shopping and try on different outfits that you wouldn't normally wear. As you do, see how this makes you feel. Imagine that rather than just putting on a different set of clothes that you are actually putting on a new persona, a new character. How does this make you feel?

8.

Telling Stories

John Killick

How do you see your life? Is it a series of different events with no real link between them – like a number of short stories, in fact? Or is it one continuously developing narrative with episodes and chapters, various characters moving in and out of it – like a novel, in fact?

If the latter, what is it that holds it together? Is it a theme or themes, or is it you, is it your personality, that makes it into a book?

If we stop to think about it the world bombards us with many different experiences, and we, as authors of our own stories, create them by fitting them into the pattern that seems to us to make most sense.

So, if we all have this need to tell stories, how does this show itself in our lives? Certainly through talk – think of the tales you hear (and just as often overhear) in the street, the pub or the café, travelling on public transport, or when visiting a friend's house. Think, too, of the long telephone calls in which people re-tell past events. But, just as we have an urge to tell other people our stories, we need even more to keep telling ourselves our stories, perhaps to reassure or try to make sense of events. The story is always being added to by new experiences – it will never be told in full. Perhaps those moments when we catch ourselves out talking aloud when alone are examples of overhearing our internal monologues. And people who live alone most of the time, mustn't they be telling their stories over and over to themselves in their heads?

How do people with dementia fit into all this? Well they are people first, and the dementia is an add-on, so they must have a need to tell their stories just like the rest of us. But maybe their need is greater than ours for this reason: since dementia is a condition which appears to undermine people's understanding and sense of being in control, to the extent that it may make them doubt where they are, and even in some instances who they are, perhaps they are literally in danger of 'losing the plot'.

The idea of being a person must be related to an individual's ability to see him or her self whole, acting and reacting in the world in a way that makes sense to them. The impulse to tell stories has to be a crucial means of maintaining this sense of identity.

One lady who had talked with me said, *'Please give me back my personality!'* She appeared to believe that she was losing her sense of self. After a number of conversations, however, in which she gradually pieced together details of her life, she began to feel more sure of her identity. She explained what she believed to be the process that had lead up to her earlier despairing request:

> *How can we begin socially because the people here don't understand my outlook and consequently have no desire to talk? I rather think that also because of my loss of memory people don't pay much attention to my conversation. And then there is my deafness. So I am left with very little social communication. I am being killed off.*

This lady could be speaking for many. She makes the point clearly that it isn't just important to be given the opportunity to talk, we must feel that we are being listened to, and what we say being taken seriously.

It is also the case that many persons with dementia are nearing the end of their lives and have much to look back upon. It is a common characteristic of older people generally that they feel the need to 'take stock' and attempt to put events into some kind of perspective. One lady said:

If you have a dream you forget about it, don't you? But I can't forget about this life that I've been through – it's with me always.

When a person feels threatened by changes in perception and the ability to make themselves understood in words, this can intensify the urgency to explore and evaluate the past. It has been our experience that some people with dementia, once given the opportunity to talk, find it difficult to stop. It is as if the ideas, incidents, feelings of a lifetime have been dammed up and begin to pour out. Some individuals are clearly telling stories (if only to themselves) before we meet them, continue with us, and carry on after we leave. Some appear to be engaged in internal monologues (and dialogues) from which we are excluded. Some of the stories we are told do not make sense to us, but clearly do to the teller; they may be mixed up in thought or language or both. But we need to entertain the possibility that though *we* may not understand what the person is saying, it makes sense to *them*.

Beth Brough (1998) in her book *Alzheimer's With Love* about her relationship with her friend Reg, who had dementia, says:

I am not proud of the fact that I was so influenced by the prevailing idea that they had 'lost their mind'. When I could not understand his speech I slipped far too readily into the myth that what was being articulated was not understandable. (Brough 1998, p.19)

She goes on to suggest that the stories Reg told were not necessarily reminiscences:

Does he know that what he is telling are tales of inner experience rather than descriptions of outer happenings? (Brough 1998, p.39)

This raises the question of whether the stories told by people with dementia are true. Well many of the stories told by anybody are unlikely wholly to be in accord with the facts. Telling a story, whether it is based on actual events or not, is a creative act, and we must expect those of people with dementia to be a mixture of truth and embellishment. A lady I spoke with remarked, *'I'm blethering, but from beneath the surface.'*

Surely our role must be to offer encouragement and create an atmosphere in which storytelling can flourish, not to be on the lookout for where a narrative may be deviating from the truth? One lady asserted her right in the following words: *'I want to make up my story for myself.'*

Most stories are told one-to-one, but I have recently experimented with Group Storytelling to good effect. It is, of course, possible to tell stories around a group, each participant adding a new strand, but I have been encouraging people to tell their own stories to others. Either I or someone with the condition acts as host. Each person in turn is invited to tell a story but the host has the key role of asking questions and helping to elicit answers from the 'guest'. Other members of the group may be invited to ask questions too. Everybody claps each storyteller when they finish. It is a remarkably affirming experience.

The leading method of group storytelling that has been developed is that by Anne Davis Basting in America. It is called 'Timeslips', and the movement offers training, a pack and a DVD. The website gives full details, including examples of stories created using the technique (see Resources list at end of the book).

Basically 'Timeslips' is a programme directed by a facilitator. It makes use of photographs carefully chosen to suggest a hidden narrative (there are examples of these too on the website). These must not be too explicit, but suggest various possible scenarios. Questions which could be asked about them include, *'Who's in the picture?'*; *'What sort of person(s) are they?'*; *'Where do they come from?'*; *'What has brought them to this place?'*; *'What happens next?'* All the answers to these and other questions from all the participants are written up by the facilitator or a scribe on a board or flipchart. No contribution is rejected on account of irrelevance; all are equally valued.

It is essential that every participant is given a copy of the picture. Pictures can be obtained from newspapers or magazines, photocopied onto card and laminated for lasting use. There is also a series of large picture-books specially created for people with dementia, and many pictures from these would be suitable; the company that produces them is called 'Pictures to Share' (see Resources list for website). Photographs of paintings can often be as potent as those of actual scenes or people. Individuals who may experience difficulty in articulating their reactions can be helped by staff, whose role is solely that of assistants – their views are excluded from the process.

The facilitator then reads out all the contributions and invites the group to add new material or change the order to make the story flow better. A title is chosen, and the complete story read out. Copies can be distributed at a later time after it has been typed up and/or exhibited on a display board. This practice can be a regular one, to which people can look forward, and to which they can become more fluent in contributing.

I have also developed a parallel process for the writing of group poems. Some of the same pictures could be used, but those with a sense of mystery seem to work best. Instead of developing a story line the object here is to capture a mood, and participants are encouraged to contribute a word or phrase or sentence which is prompted by their emotional reaction to the picture. Any attempt to offer rhymes is discouraged: that would add a layer of difficulty and perhaps distortion: this has to be a free-verse effort.

Both of these approaches can be initiated by anyone with a minimum of expertise but a maximum of enthusiasm. They are inclusive rather than exclusive, and can benefit a wide range of people. Necessarily the results are less personal than individual stories and poems but offer real opportunities for the experience of enjoyment in taking part and shared pride in the result.

TRY-OUTS

Think about what happened yesterday. Make a list of all the occasions you told a story yourself or listened to someone else's. This can include conversations across a meal-table, meetings in a pub or café, a shop, an office, the street; also telephone (mobile) conversations, emails, tweets, blogs, etc. Choose one of these and try to assess its significance for yourself or for another person. Find a photograph album or a set of photographs on a disk or stored on your computer. Choose a series or an individual one that suggests a narrative, and write that story.

9.

Conversations in Paint

Claire Craig

Mary picks up the brush and makes a mark on the paper. Bold, deliberate. I reciprocate with a fainter line. She sits for a second momentarily distracted by a conversation happening in another part of the care home and I wonder if she has had enough for today. I say her name and she looks at her hand holding the brush almost in surprise. I make another mark, a circle this time and she looks on and smiles directly at me. Then, dipping her brush in the red she begins, head down, absorbed in the process of creating shape and form, her brush moving first this way and then that. She begins to sing. In front of my eyes a scene emerges – a field of red and black. 'My brothers never returned from the war,' she says simply, a statement of fact and then adds, 'it feels a long way from home.'

Visual art is a statement, an expression of something about how we feel and who we are, conveyed through colour, line or form. If art is seen as an unfolding story rather than simply as an end product, as a conversation or reflection rather than an exercise in producing an accurate depiction of a scene you can quickly see how the canvas becomes a meeting place where relationships can develop and self-esteem and identity can flourish. This requires us to think about the visual arts in their broadest sense embracing all forms including simple mark making, paper marbling and doodling as well as painting and drawing.

One of the greatest strengths of this media is the breadth it offers in terms of engagement and communication on many different levels. The person may talk about the image-making process for instance, or the end result. Art also operates very much on a non-verbal level and communication may take place on the page through the art. The messages transmitted through the images remain long after the art-making process has ended. An artist, on seeing an exhibition of paintings by people with dementia said:

I was told that a number of these artists were unable to communicate. They often are reclusive and confused. Their paintings however are clear, straightforward, richly coloured and above all communicative. (Jenny and Oropeza 1993, p.80)

The final works can challenge our perceptions in relation to who people with dementia are and what people think and feel. Visual art can also embody something of our personality. Selly Jenny captures this in her description of Helen, a person with dementia:

Her wonderful sense of humour is shown in her painting and her description of herself, 'just call me Alice in Wonderland.' The bold strokes of this sketch are a contrast to the shy, small person who is Helen. She paints with a self-assurance that reflects back and gives us a peek at the competent woman that she once was. (Jenny and Oropeza 1993)

The aim then is to offer choice rather than restrict or limit what a person can achieve and it will be necessary for you to think carefully about the materials you share. Good quality paper and art materials are a must (suggestions are included at the end of this chapter). I am dismayed when I see visual art confined to crayons and colouring books which not only carry powerful childlike connotations, limiting the quality of the work produced but stifle any form of self-expression reducing the creative act to following instructions and matching colours. Art is freedom and individuality not conformity and repetition.

People paint and draw for lots of different reasons. Some individuals I have worked alongside have painted because it has been a treasured hobby, or a skill they want to develop, others because they want to achieve a pleasing end result or to create something to give to a family member or friend. For yet others it has been a much needed outlet for self-expression; anger, sadness, frustration have all found release and been communicated through marks on the page. This will in some way shape the types of art activity that you might want to share with the person. The central pages of this book includes images created by people with dementia that illustrate something of the breadth of the opportunities it can provide.

Many approaches to sharing the visual arts exist. Some of these tap into the inherent quality of art to tell a story/exploiting the way we paint from experience/paint what we know best. The programme 'Memories in the Making' would be a good example of this. Here, artists work alongside the person and help them use the visual media to recreate a memory so that through the paint they are able to tell their story. Emphasis is placed on the social dimension of the experience so that *'class sessions are still very much social events in which no-one works alone or must 'risk' making something from beginning to end, by themselves'* (Jenny and Oropeza 1993, p.47).

'Creating together' is another technique of working alongside a person in the making of joint pieces of art work. This has grown from the recognition that some people, because of their dementia, experience difficulties in initiating movement and taking the first step to engage in creative activities (Baines 2007). It also acknowledges that visual art has a strong social dimension, lending itself to group as well as individual interactions. For instance group painting, visual mosaics (see next page) where the artwork is a cumulative effort offers opportunities to connect people, promoting a sense of togetherness and community. Of equal value is the process of painting alongside someone, working independently but in the same creative space. Where people with dementia have painted alongside their partner this has very much been about relationship, time together and a connection that transcends the physical and is more intuitive or spiritual.

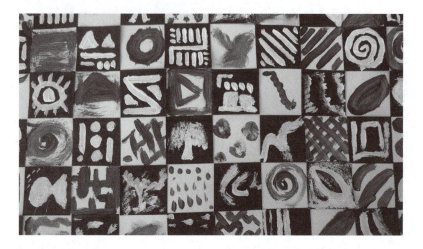

Marks made with white paint on a black background and marks made with black paint on a white background present a striking visual mosaic

I personally like to begin by offering the person space to gain a feel for art, perhaps looking through art books, exploring different styles and possible themes for painting. This can lead to all sorts of interesting conversations. One person I was sharing this activity with seized upon a painting by Klimt and tapping the image said, *'look at that, he's tickling her fancy but she's not sure about him. It's in her eyes.'* She went on to create an image called 'lost love,' an allegory of her own relationship.

I also like to offer the person the opportunity to explore different kinds of media. At its simplest level this can be something as straightforward as sitting with the person with a large sheet of paper looking at the effect that different art materials make. Another activity that works well is to 'take a line for a walk' where you begin by making a mark on a sheet of paper and then invite others to continue the line, taking it in whatever direction and in whatever colour or shape it may choose to go. Both offer important clues and cues in terms of what works for the person. For instance, how they are able to hold and manipulate the media, whether the impermanence and control offered by a pencil, for example, suits them better than the fluidity of paint and whether

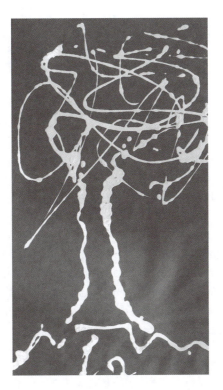

Taking a line for a walk

there are textures they find particularly difficult (e.g. some people find the texture of pastels or chalks unpleasant).

Engaging with the materials in this way can also help to build confidence and take away the pressure of immediately being expected to produce 'something'. It introduces the idea of creative play where the artistic media become the vehicle for self-expression, a journey to wherever you choose to go. Painting to music would be a good example of this where a piece of music is played and the person responds to the music through the art media – sweeping brush strokes, sharp dots, zig-zags and patterns so the final image becomes a visual representation of the music and the mood, rhythm, story or feeling it conveys. Here, the focus is on the expressive qualities of the materials.

The idea of turning one thing into something else can be helpful in terms of releasing creative flow as is the case with impermanent art. Here art is seen as improvisation and imagination. The person is offered an assortment of objects (buttons, wool, cotton, sequins, leaves) anything that can be found to hand and invited to arrange these on a piece of card or fabric. Choice, decision making and creative play are strong features of this activity. During one memorable session, Albert, a person with dementia, set a fabulous challenge of creating a portrait from a single piece of string. Everyone on the ward took part and the results were dramatic and insightful since even these crude materials had captured something about the subject whether it was the shape of the face or the angle of the glasses. We photographed the end results thereby transforming these impermanent works into something more lasting. Painting beyond an image where the artist paints 'what lies beyond' a picture or a postcard, moving beyond the parameters can also be exceptionally freeing.

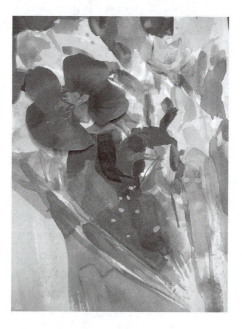

An example of painting beyond the image

Clearly much depends on the person and what they hope to achieve from the interaction. Some individuals you will work alongside may come to you with the expressed aim of wanting to build their skills in painting and drawing. In these instances it can be very helpful to work with community artists or individuals who are skilled in teaching techniques in art making. Betty Edwards (1993) in her book, *Drawing on the Right Side of the Brain* also describes a number of methods we have found to be particularly useful. The final presentation of the work is important. A cardboard mount or a frame, the act of naming the piece giving it a title finishes the work and gives the image and its artist the respect they deserve.

The visual arts present people with dementia a palette of opportunities. Given all that they offer it is unsurprising that people with dementia have described art as, '*more important than eating or sleeping*' (Grace, a person with dementia in Baines 2007, p.10). Patricia Baines (2007) recounts one interaction where a person with dementia turned to her and said, '*This is very important for us. You should come again*' (Baines 2007, p.13) leading her to reflect that, '*The power of image making is that it allows those with dementia to express herself or himself in ways that are satisfying and communicate with others*' (Baines 2007, p.40).

Yet in spite of the many opportunities it offers, of all the creative art forms we describe in this book the visual arts can be one of the most difficult to get to grips with. This is because before you even begin working with people with dementia you will have a whole range of preconceptions in terms of what the visual arts are, what constitutes good art and bad art and this will be infused with your personal experiences of art making at school and college. As a consequence this area is fraught with emotion since art does not conform, is not predictable and challenges the norm. It is precisely this quality that makes it so valuable in the context of people with dementia and enables it to be the medium for change and growth that it is. I end this chapter with the words of Robert Henri who said:

When the artist is alive in any person, whatever his kind of work may be, he becomes an inventive, searching, daring, self-expressive creature. He becomes interesting to other people. He disturbs, upsets, enlightens, and opens up ways for a better understanding. Where those who are not artists are trying to close the book he opens it and shows there are still more pages possible. (Robert Henri, The Art Spirit in Edwards 1993, p.6)

What to include in your art box

Art books, postcards, calendars, recycled greetings cards.

Pens, pencils, eraser.

Glue sticks.

Assortment of paints and good quality paint brushes.

Pastels.

Water colour paper, tissue paper.

Backing board (for framing images).

TRY-OUTS

About you and painting: do you paint? Have you ever painted? If yes, what do you gain from this? If no, what stops you from painting? What would you need to enable you to paint?

What words spring to mind when you think about painting and drawing...

Describe a good experience and a bad experience you have had at school in relation to painting or drawing. Has this impacted on you now?

Imagine that you have been asked to share a piece of art you have made? How would this feel? Who would you feel comfortable sharing this work with? Is there anyone you wouldn't want to share this with? If not, why?

Go to your local art gallery. Find a piece of art that you love. Find a piece of art that you hate or that angers you.

Try to work out what it is about the art that provokes this response.

What is the purpose of visual art? Is it to challenge? To inspire? To add something that is aesthetically beautiful to the world? To create an emotional connection?

What do you think you can learn about the artist and how they were feeling when looking at a work of art?

10.

Playing with Mud

Ceramics and Clay

Claire Craig

Clay is the type of material that seems to evoke a love/hate relationship. I can recall all too clearly the first time I invited a person with dementia to make something, placing a lump of clay in her hands. The reaction was immediate. She literally threw it across the room, and with a voice and look filled with contempt said, *'Don't you ever ask me to play with mud again!'*

Clay is incredibly tactile. For some individuals its texture, temperature and the residue it leaves on the surfaces it encounters is too much. Comments from people with dementia have included, *'it's dirty,' 'it's slimy,' 'it's cold like a snake'*. Yet for others its malleability, substance and consistency make it the creative medium of choice and they find that the prospect of playing with mud is quite appealing.

For one thing the process of engaging with and working the material can be extremely physical. Wedging is the name given to preparing the raw clay so that it has the correct consistency for working and doesn't contain any air bubbles. There are various techniques that include kneading, slapping and throwing the raw material, usually on a canvas (hessian is perfect) or plaster surface.

It is usually performed standing and is an excellent way to work off pent-up energy or frustration. It is often quite a loud affair, but can provide a powerful outlet for emotions. Jock, a person I worked with who became extremely depressed and angry after being diagnosed with dementia would frequently just turn up at the occupational therapy department with the express purpose of wedging. It gave him permission to work through strong emotions in an environment where it was acceptable to do this.

Wedging is a very physical process and is not appropriate where individuals are physically frail. The starting point for these interactions is to offer small balls of pre-wedged clay for working. It is interesting to see where this process leads. Some of the most enjoyable sessions have been where a group of us have sat around the table, clay balls in hand, pinching, smoothing, shaping the material, trusting the process and waiting in expectation to see where this leads and what the material becomes.

There is much to be said for 'listening to the material'. This immediately takes the pressure off feeling that it is necessary to produce anything in particular, offering permission to enjoy the sensory journey seeing where the clay leads. Sometimes conversation focuses on the texture of the material: *This feels as smooth as a baby's bottom'* has been an opening line used on many occasions. It has also led to some really interesting results. One person broke off pieces of clay and rolled these into tiny balls. The title she gave to her work was 'Spilling Out'. Animals have featured strongly in many pieces – one person made a model of her cat, another the snake he had adopted in India. 'Frightened Little Bunny' was the title of another work. Food often emerges as a theme. Sometimes the clay simply remains as a shape – 'Cactus' was one memorable work and another where two lumps of clay were broken apart the artist tellingly named the piece 'Ripped in Two'.

In all these instances the clay has offered a means to learn about who someone is, giving shape to fears, hopes and dreams or simply providing space for friendship in an environment of making. The great strength is the three-dimensional nature of the medium, allowing the person to mould and model the material and then step back, move around the piece and see it from different perspectives, reflecting on what has been produced. Where individuals or groups have found the act of holding or touching the material too difficult they have taken on the role of 'director' in the process instructing me how to manipulate the clay into the shape they desire.

Another way of working with the medium I have found to be particularly successful includes instances where the clay has been rolled out (using two wooden girders) and then cut into squares. Individuals have then spent time decorating and personalising these tiles which have later adorned rooms or been given as presents to family members. In one setting a magnificent group piece was created where each person contributed a separate tile representing something about a given month and these had then been mounted in the foyer of the building. This offered a very powerful statement as to the skills and talents of individuals living there. Beth Meyer Arnold, an artist in America, has reported great success in a programme offering people with dementia the opportunity to make and decorate their own tiles and masks from clay (Basting 2003, p.17) and also suggests that men respond particularly well to working in 3-D.

One of the biggest challenges in terms of the material is the cost of the activity. A number of care environments have invested in kilns and drying rooms or have had these donated. Nonetheless the raw material isn't cheap and the cost of firing materials in the kiln is extremely expensive. In some settings we have been able to team up with local colleges or schools who have offered their services, but the challenge then is how to transport the pieces.

One solution is to investigate alternatives. For instance there are a range of materials that have the same consistency as clay but do not need to be fired: air drying clay, for example, is a good substitute. If the focus is on jewellery making, then Fimo would be the material of choice. This still has the same consistency of clay and can be rolled into balls and beads, but it arrives in ready-made colours and can be baked in the oven. With all these materials it is important to check toxicity and to take the necessary measures to ensure that the activity is safe for the person to engage in. The other possibility to investigate would be mosaic where the focus is more on using or re-using ceramic and other materials.

The principles of mosaic are very simple. Fundamentally the process involves sticking the mosaic materials to the object and then filling the spaces between the pieces of decorative material with grout to form a continuous resilient surface (Matthews 2003, p.21). It is possible to mosaic just about anything. The one thing to be aware of is that the surface needs to be clean and dry before you begin and if the surface is porous it needs to be sealed with diluted PVA before the decoration is applied (Matthews 2003). Mosaic offers the person an opportunity to express something of who they are and to make their mark on the outside or inside environments where they live. It is an extremely expressive, creative activity, offering many opportunities for choice, decision making, building pattern and having fun, although it can also contain a sense of order. There is a very powerful clip on *Art for the Person's Sake*, a film about Sandwell Third Age Arts (a project John was involved in) where a person at quite an advanced stage of dementia who appears to find it very difficult to settle approaches a mosaic activity, again and again, choosing tiles and pressing them onto the surface. Clearly she finds the activity extremely pleasurable, sitting for short periods of time, completely focused.

Mosaic can be undertaken as an individual activity or as a group effort. Ceramic pots, planters and indoor picture frames have all offered excellent projects. In one hospital setting the artist in residence had used mosaic to aid way-finding in the grounds surrounding the assessment ward for people with dementia. The end pieces offered an immediate talking point and their slightly raised surfaces and tactile nature offered an excellent way to involve people with sensory impairment.

It is possible to mosaic with just about anything – pebbles, shells, glass beads, mirror. In the days before health and safety we would use broken ceramics! However, it is now possible to buy ready-made strips of ceramic squares with smooth edges which are very easy to work with.

Ceramics in whatever guise it takes offer a range of opportunities for people with dementia. From 'playing with mud' through to crafting mosaic this medium has many different qualities that individuals can use as a means of self-expression and exploration. The added strength is that the end pieces have a permanence, a certain depth, weight and substance to them that says, 'I'm here' and cannot be ignored.

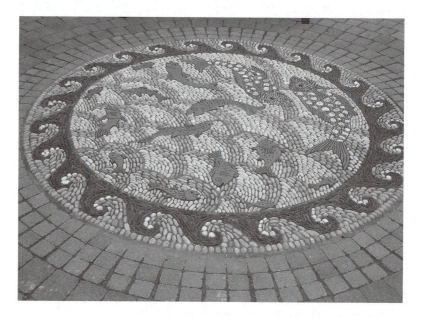

An example of a mosaic made from stones at the Iris Murdoch Centre

In the art box

Air drying clay.

Fimo.

Spoons, forks, different tools that could make an impression on the material.

Pieces of hessian.

Pre-bought mosaic tiles, a tub of grout.

Aprons and old shirts (very important to protect clothes), nail file (to remove clay from under nails).

TRY-OUTS

Spend a day being aware of textures – the mug you hold, the feel of bathroom tiles under foot. Are there any textures you find particularly pleasant or difficult?

See if you can track down examples of mosaic in your local community – churches may have some or other faith centres. What stories do the mosaics tell? What do you notice about the colours and textures used?

11.

Working with the Hard Stuff
Stone, Wood, Metal and Glass

Claire Craig

You may be surprised to see a chapter pertaining to stone, wood, metal and glass in a book about creativity and communication for persons with dementia. The materials are expensive, can be challenging to work with and require the use of specialist tools or equipment. Consequently it could easily be assumed that such work is highly specialised and out of the reach of most of us. However, John and I have both known people with dementia for whom working with the 'hard stuff' has been a source of great pleasure, mastery and enjoyment and as such a chapter dedicated to this rightfully takes its place in our book.

First, let me begin by considering the appeal of these materials. Stone, wood, metal and glass are solid and possess an air of permanence which means they will remain long after other organic materials such as fabric and paper have faded and decayed. This has been important for some people for whom the idea of leaving a mark, a legacy for future generations has mattered, something to say, 'I was here.'

The materials carry weight, suggesting strength and gravitas. The daughter of one person with dementia whose father was building an igloo type structure from lumps of firewood in the back room insightfully reflected, *'We all know what he is doing. He is letting us know that this is his home, his territory, making sure we can still see him.'* This has been true for other people for whom the materials have made a statement and a sort of inverse process has taken place whereby the more a person's confidence or sense of being heard has diminished, the bolder the artwork has become, a projection and extension of self.

If the materials carry weight they also demand involvement and engagement – shaping, moving, positioning; placing the person in control. This can offer a sense of mastery. Christophe Grillet is a person who took up sculpture following a diagnosis of dementia. His wife describes how the process of learning to carve was *'a difficult and emotional journey, but it helped his self-esteem and feelings that he could still be creative.'* Christophe has exhibited his work nationally, leading to a number of paid commissions (we have included an image of one of his works 'Guard Dog' in the colour section of the book).

However, whilst gaining such mastery can be 'a difficult and emotional journey', people with dementia have also spoken of the value of working within the boundaries imposed by the qualities of the material, for instance the malleability of the metal, the fragility of the glass. Moreover because you begin with the raw material there is always the sense you are beginning with something as opposed to nothing so there is a ready-made starting point whether this is the shape of the stone, the texture of the glass, the angle of the wood and the challenge is to explore, understand and respond to this.

The process is above all extremely tactile. This might be immediately apparent when sanding wood, or polishing stone, however, it is equally true of working with metal and glass. For instance artist Steve Davidson has exploited the qualities of textured glass in his work with people with dementia. The colour, shape, translucence and feel of the final pieces of stained glass individuals have created with his support and direction are testament to the range of sensory qualities this material offers.

Making stained glass is a specialist and complex process and the involvement of artists confident in working with the medium is important to ensure that this is both a positive and safe experience. Steve and his wife, occupational therapist Christine Davidson, fully involve and support individuals at each stage of the process whether this is in drawing up the original designs, choosing the pieces of glass or placing these in the final configuration they will take. Each person works within their own comfort zone. However, if such resources are not available there are other, less specialist ways of working with this material. I have been part of a number of arts projects, for example, where people with dementia have engaged in glass painting taking jars, bottles and picture frames and transforming these into beautiful works of art using glass paints purchased from a local art shop.

The same can be said of all these media – sculpture, woodcarving and metal work are best supported by artists skilled in understanding the media with access to the specialist materials required, although simpler variations based around the theme can be just as effective. For instance our friend James McKillop has dementia. He is exceptionally skilled at polishing stones and I have spent a happy afternoon in the comfort of his kitchen learning from James how to do this. I have certainly nowhere the number of commissions James has received for his work, although the pieces adorn my home and desk at work. This would be a perfect activity for people who want to work with stone but who may not have access to the materials required for sculpture. Similarly I have known a number of men with dementia who have relished the opportunity to work with wood, sanding pieces until they are smooth and pebble like. For some individuals it has offered an outlet for pent-up emotion and frustration, for others the familiarity of the materials has tapped into memories relating to previous roles, offering mastery and building self-esteem. This has particularly been the case with men who spent a lifetime working in the steelworks or on construction sites where the need to build has been innate. For people such as Ernest whose response to all other art forms was one of distaste: *'naaaw it's woman's work, what do you take me for lass?'* the opportunity to work with wood offers an acceptable meaningful activity.

For more ambitious projects – and I would suggest that you think big – artist networks, local colleges and art departments within universities are all useful. I can certainly call to mind people with dementia I have worked alongside who have attended courses with partners or family members and as a result of this process developed shared hobbies. One of the most memorable was a person I recently met who has just returned from a weekend in the Lake District where he and his wife attended a glass blowing course. He struggled to communicate verbally although his voice was bubbling with excitement as he shared image after image of the experience. I regularly go to workshops offered by a local sculpture park that have included the construction of willow withies, life-sized sculptures made from recycled materials and I have attempted wood-carving. These themed days are held in outside spaces and would offer a perfect opportunity for people with dementia and their families to be involved in a process of making together. On a personal level I have really enjoyed the opportunity of working with artists and learning about the materials. Above all, the experience has taught me that part of the appeal of working with the 'hard stuff' is the relationship developed during the process of making. In part this is about the bond formed between artist and object since the process engages you physically, mentally and emotionally. However, in part it also refers to the relationship forged between artist and student since in my experience the process of making and mastering these materials is one of partnership, of co-creation. This sentiment is echoed in the work of Caroline Twist, activity co-ordinator and Dr Jayne Wallace, researcher. Caroline and Jayne are both artist jewellers and have worked extensively with people with dementia. Caroline uses metals such as brass and copper and Jayne works with a broad range of materials including metal, wood, cloth and digital media. However, both focus on the potential of the process to support the individual's identity and sense of self.

Caroline for instance has developed a way of transforming reminiscences into tangible objects, beautiful pieces of jewellery comprising of people's words using her skills in metalwork to create three-dimensional representations of these memories and in doing so build relationships and reinforce the person's sense of identity. Each piece is informed by and made alongside the person. Similarly Jayne very much sees:

> *jewellery as a symbol of self, as something that becomes a witness to our experiences, as a signifier of aspects of identity and inter-personal relationships, as a conduit to transport us to other times, places and people, and as a receptacle for our feelings of that associated 'other'.* (www.digitaljewellery.com)

She involves the person with dementia in the design process with the goal of making digital jewellery objects for the individual and the people close to them to help support the maintenance of self and personhood. She describes a recent project working with Gillian, a person with dementia and her husband John:

> *The pieces are products of Gillian, John and us — not of us as designers reacting to them. Co-creativity is a powerful element — people invest in the pieces and can continue to create them over time — the co-creativity gives them the permission to get involved — so the process is less a 'them and us' situation it is something more democratised and shared.* (www.digitaljewellery.com)

In both instances the focus is on 'creating together' and perhaps this is the strength of working with all these materials since they invite this type of collaboration and depend very much on shared relationship where the final pieces represent a journey travelled together.

Working with the hard stuff is not for everyone. However, it is for some. That is the point and for this reason the potential of making with wood, stone, metal or glass in whatever guise should not be overlooked.

TRY-OUTS

Collect a range of objects made of different materials (e.g. a glass jar, a stone, a metal thimble). Take each one in turn and explore these with your eyes closed. What do you feel? Do you have any particular likes and dislikes in relation to the materials? Share these objects with a person with dementia, note their response. What do you think is the story behind their making?

Visit a sculpture exhibition, preferably one that encourages some form of interaction with the pieces. See if you can identify pieces that you make a particular 'connection' with.

Investigate opportunities in your locality for courses in wood and metalwork. If formal courses do not exist see if you can arrange a visit to an artist's workshop.

12.

Textured Journeys
Exploring the Potential of Textiles

Claire Craig

Right then lass who's got them whisty bits? Is that you Florrie? Put them down flat… Thas never seen flat. And them others. Right they go't other way. Do we roll yet…right not yet, we need soap and water. Now we roll. I love this part. Separates girls from 't boys.

It's a vivid memory of a session in the hospital where I worked. There were four of us gathered around a table on the ward making felt. Jack had taken control of the process. He had been referred because he was low in mood, struggling to come to terms with dementia, lashing out, venting his frustration on others. Felting for Jack though was the ultimate activity. It offered him an outlet, an opportunity to be in control and restore some of the fragile self-esteem that dementia had taken away. The activity worked on a number of levels. There was the making of the felt for one and all that entailed, the choice, the decision making, placing of one colour against another to create the design. However, beyond this there were the sensory qualities of the end result. I remember this distinctly because Jack and I worked at sewing the squares together (and there were a great number of these) into a blanket.

This became a real talking point and was something he carried with him from place to place. It became a means to signify where he was sitting and a source of comfort as he sat, blanket on knee stroking it as though it were a long-lost cat.

The creative potential of textiles is often overlooked, yet it should not be underestimated. For one thing textiles work on so many different levels: felting, weaving, patchwork, silk painting, working with wool, even the dyeing of fabrics provide the opportunity for choice, decision making, self-expression and have an added value of tapping into previously valued roles spanning back to an era of make-do and mend. These activities literally formed part of the fabric of everyday life where mothers passed their skills to daughters and the garments created were rites of passage: the first pair of bootees, the first matinee jacket were treasured heirlooms, acts of love.

I have worked alongside individuals who have recently been diagnosed with dementia where the element of 'making' has been particularly important. Yet by the same token people who have lived with dementia for some time have been able to engage just as fully through the sensory component of the media. Working with textiles is also inherently sociable and the act of taking part in rag-rugging or quilting where everyone sits and works together has inspired feelings of connectedness, fun and friendship, prompting participants to share stories whilst also promoting a sense of shared ownership in the final piece.

Indeed, knitting and crochet have recently undergone a renaissance with knitting circles being very much in vogue amongst the twenty-something age group, offering great scope as an intergenerational activity, positioning the person with dementia as expert in sharing skills and techniques.

This means that everyone can be involved. The inclusive nature of the medium also extends to time since many of the activities can be undertaken in short bursts – put down and then picked up later which makes this ideal to share with people who find it difficult to concentrate.

Within textiles, more marked than other creative media, is the creativity continuum. At one end are activities that involve a level of technical ability and familiarity with specific techniques. Knitting, crochet and embroidery would be good examples of this category offering space for creativity, but within certain parameters. At the other end of the spectrum are those activities that offer more opportunities for expression. It is on this part of the spectrum that the chapter focuses.

The starting point always begins with an invitation to explore materials – yarns, silk scarves, raw wool fibres, fleece squares – a fabric feast. Sometimes the materials are enough, prompting discussion or reminiscence. During one session a person grabbed one of the threads from a ball of wool someone was holding and called out: *'It's like a giant umbilical cord. We're all connected,'* and another person said, *'See that tangled mess – well that's how my brain feels – but it is really beautiful.'* Balls of blue or pink wool are often seized upon, lovingly held and nurtured as memories of children or childhood are shared. There is also the opportunity for sharing and humour. One older person from a knitting project described by Fiona Rutherford recounted:

> *Before I was married I knitted my boyfriend a bathing costume, trunks in grey wool. He was from Newcastle and swam in galas for Northumberland, but when he got into the baths they went wide. It was a bit embarrassing. He said, 'never knit me a pair of them again'.* (Rutherford and Burns 2008, p.13)

We have seen people at quite an advanced point in their dementia spontaneously pick up balls of wool and begin to finger knit or hold out their hands, in anticipation to begin wool-winding. Others have seized upon materials and engaged in impromptu drama sessions where chiffon pieces have become wedding dresses or where scarves have become props for exotic dances.

There is no denying that the materials have a strong expressive quality. The image on page 87 is a photograph of an abstract piece of art built up by sculpting or layering different fabrics and was created by Rozena, a person with dementia. Rozena spends much of her time sitting in a wheelchair. Her muscles are wasted which means that she doesn't have much control over her head, so she more or less sits with her head twisted to one side. Although she doesn't speak, she is incredibly communicative and very creative. Touch is particularly important and one of the ways she makes her needs known. We begin, sitting together exploring the different fabrics: silk scarves, coloured handkerchiefs, balls of wool. I introduce a wooden tray with a slightly raised rim which effectively acts as a canvas. I show Rozena different fabrics that could form a background. Sometimes she takes hold of ones that she doesn't like and throws them to the floor. Sometimes when I offer her a choice, she does this using eye pointing or touch and so the process continues, building up layer after layer of fabric, placing the materials quite deliberately on the wooden canvas. When she has finished I frame the final piece with cardboard made from backing board and she sits tray on her lap, stroking the fabrics, sensing the three-dimensional image she has created.

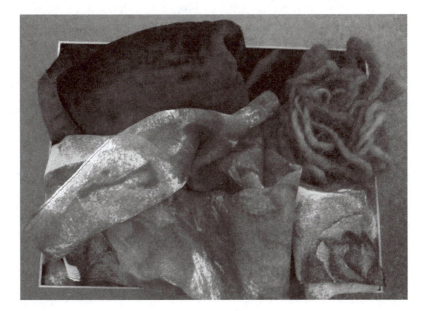

A fabric image

Felting is another exceptionally versatile and expressive medium that uses a similar principle to the one just described. It involves building up layers of raw material (merino wool) which are then fused together by breaking down the fibres with a solution of warm, soapy water and exerting friction either by rubbing or by placing the fibres between netting and rolling until they interlock and a piece of felt is formed. An example of this can be found in the colour section. The process works well when undertaken individually or as a group. Warm soapy water and wool offer a sensory experience reminiscent of washday and sessions tend to be lively events although some care needs to be taken. The process of rolling the fabric to break down the fibres can be a good outlet for pent-up energy; there is also something quite rhythmic to the process, described by one person as 'rocking' that can feel quite calming and relaxing.

Weaving, with its emphasis on rhythm and order can also be quite relaxing. During a training session about the arts a person immediately identified this quality. She said, *'I started to weave when Mum first developed dementia and now she joins me and we sit together. It is something we both enjoy. It is our time and I treasure all these pieces because we have made them and they are part of us.'* Ginty Fay describes a similar story in relation to her husband, Bob who developed frontal lobe dementia. Beginning with rug-making their interests broadened to encompass weaving and tapestry. The benefits she describes are wide-ranging, including the alleviation of stress, increased self-esteem, enjoyment, the development of a shared activity they can both enjoy which brings them both into touch with other people in the wider community (Fay 1995).

It is possible to weave with just about anything. Philomena Wynne has developed a technique called wild weaving which takes as its frame bleached sticks which act as a hanger, on which the person can weave a range of materials including wool, feathers, paper, beads, pieces of paper. Described by the artist as, 'like painting with textiles' the process affords the person a great deal of freedom (www.wildweaving.co.uk).

Weaving can therefore be an exceptionally expressive medium through which it is possible to 'weave emotion' each piece of ribbon or yarn representing a different feeling depicted by texture or colour, or create woven stories (much in the same way that Persian carpets often contained the secret name of its creator's lover represented by different threads). Similar ideas can be used within rag-rugging (or pogging as it known in some parts of the country). This is such a simple process which uses hessian as the base, rags or pieces of fabric cut into 2-inch strips as the threads, and the tool is a wooden peg with a pointed end which is used to make a hole and push the fabric through.

Within all these processes the final piece is always a tangible reminder of the textured journey you have travelled together in their creation and your evolving relationship. These textured journeys are remarkable and represent points of connections, meeting places. There is great potential here for drawing people together. For instance in Hilary Lee's project 'Weaving cherished memories and childhood dreams', people with dementia shared their skills in rug-making with schoolchildren to create a giant tapestry, in which their memories were interwoven with the hopes and dreams of the students (Lee 2006). A similar project by Judith Perry (1997) in Warwickshire which involved the design and production of three wall-hangings emphasised the value of offering young people the opportunity to work and learn from people with dementia.

Over time you will come to experience the different qualities of fibres and fabrics and discover ways to tap into these. Weaving is all about rhythm and order, felting is energy and temperature, rag rugging is pattern and texture. However, perhaps the strength of all these media is this inherent quality to bring people together. The processes of weaving the threads, or fusing the fibres, finding ways to join them to create pattern and substance is somehow mirrored in the lives of those taking part so that they too become intertwined, joined through engaging in this shared experience and learning about each other.

In the arts box

Pieces of fabric, thread, string, ribbon, old clothes.

Pieces of hessian and felt-tipped pens (to mark out a pattern).

Scissors.

Merino wool (for felting).

Sheets of plastic, bubblewrap.

Knitting needles.

Crochet hook.

TRY-OUTS

Seek out different fabrics – items of clothing, scarves, upholstery, rugs, wall-hangings, cushions and bedding. Spend a few moments exploring their textures. Are there any fabrics you are drawn to particularly? What attracts you to these: is it their colour, their feel, their weight or texture? Do some fabrics remind you of particular events or periods of your life? For instance towelling nappies, silk taffeta, flannelette, denim, starched shirts? Can you identify particular memories associated with particular items of clothing?

Does what you wear influence how you behave? Try wearing different items of clothing. What is the effect of wearing a different colour or a different texture?

Fold a sheet with a colleague or a partner. As you do think of an emotion and try folding the sheet in this manner. For instance you could choose to express anger or joy or enthusiasm. Without telling your partner, see if they can sense the emotion through the fabric. Compare experiences.

Do you have any texture likes and dislikes? Some people for instance either like or particularly dislike cotton wool or certain types of wool or go cold at the texture of some silks.

13.

Between Memory and Imagination

Collage and Life-Story Work[1]

Claire Craig

Working with paper spans the fields of collage, papier-mâchè, quilling, origami and decoupage which are all art forms within their own right. The medium of paper has a number of immediate advantages: cost for one, the sensory component of the materials another and the three dimensionality that can be achieved when creating structures, offering something to hold and to physically share with others. It is also exceptionally accessible. People who frequently shy away from other forms of creative media can feel less inhibited when invited to work and play with paper. This can be for a number of reasons: the material is familiar, can be easily manipulated, the activities tend to be quite structured, tapping into notions of recycling and reusing material. There is also much to be said for starting with one set of materials and turning them into something else rather than being overwhelmed with a blank sheet of paper and the endless options this presents.

---

1 This title is inspired by Gibson in her description of life-story work as using the interplay between memory and imagination

For the purposes of this book I have chosen to focus on ways of working with paper in relation to life-story work concentrating predominantly but not exclusively on the use of collage. In doing this I certainly don't intend to imply that collage should only ever be autobiographical in nature or that life-story work should predominantly focus on collage, and to this end I have included a chapter at the end of the book illustrating a broader approach to this important area.

Collage describes a technique of cutting, shaping, arranging and sticking down pieces of paper, photographs, and other objects to a supporting surface. The starting point is in the selection of materials: copies of photographs, images and words taken from magazines, objects that will be incorporated into the image. I once overheard a person with dementia telling her friend, *'You can use any old junk, just so long as it's yours.'*

The next phase is deciding on the layout of the materials and trimming these to size. Opportunities for choice and decision making here abound. The images take on a giant jigsaw puzzle-like quality. One of the best descriptions of this was by a colleague who had observed an interaction and recalled that it was like, *'Two people looking at a box of chocolates drooling over their contents and deciding which to eat first.'*

Karen Jarvis (2001) has written an excellent guide that includes valuable tips such as placing the larger and more important items of photographs in the foreground and gradually reducing the size of images towards the back and creating depth by placing brighter or darker colours in the foreground. The final stage is gluing the images and objects in place. Some people we have worked alongside have chosen to use a mixed media approach, painting the background or embellishing different images. Either way each collage that is made is a unique piece of artwork, reflecting something of who the person is and what is important.

This simple process yields striking results. If you are in any doubt look at the work of Ray Maloney who took up collage following his diagnosis of dementia. The works comprise of layers of acrylic paint, images from magazines and words that express something of the impact of the condition on his life and articulate his feelings about this. The end pieces are powerful and communicative, constituting a visual embodiment of his experiences of living with dementia (for an example of one of Ray's collages please see the colour photograph of his work, 'Safe Haven' contained in the colour section of the book). Ray's work illustrates beautifully how collage allows people with dementia to express what is important in ways that are not dependent on words. Jarvis describes it in this way:

> *People with dementia often have little control over many aspects of their life. Decisions are usually made for them. Collages are a unique, individualised approach to each person. They can enhance self-esteem and reinforce 'identity'.* (Jarvis 2001, p.2)

She emphasises the value of this medium in relation to both life-story work and reminiscence. This reference to life-story work has resonances here. Life-story work can be defined as 'aspects of someone's life that reinforces the person rather than the dementia.' (Murphy 1994). It can be seen as both a process and a product and is quite distinct from the more in-depth, psychological intervention of life review which focuses on coming to terms with life experiences and resolving past conflicts (Bruce and Schweitzer 2008, p.170)

Over the last few years there has been a growing recognition of the value of life-story work for people with dementia (McKeown *et al.* 2006, Moos and Bjorn 2006, Pietrukowicz and Johnson 1991) and a number of excellent accounts describing how to facilitate the process exist (Murphy 1994; Murphy 1995; Shipway 1999) including those in the main references. The emphasis of this work is very much on identity, dignity, relationship and personhood (Clarke *et al.* 2003; Coker 1998; Edwards and Chapman 2004). The best life-story work offers a picture of the person in the here and now. Less useful are those stories that are created as a checklist (likes, dislikes, name of family, previous job) offering static two-dimensional historical accounts of who the person was 10, 20 or even 30 years ago. A good life-story is not a one-off event but an ongoing journey with the individual, a dynamic portrait of the person which accurately reflects the changing nature of who they are, where the past is a part of this, and a means to give context to the present.

Collage and other paper-based arts media offer tangible ways for people with dementia to express and tell their individual stories in ways that are not dependent on words (Carr *et al.* 2009). These stories exist on multiple levels and may be told through the materials the person uses, the images they include, through the words woven into the collage or the ongoing story of its creation. The great strength of this approach is that the final pieces offer a great immediacy as well as communicating something of the multi-layered and complex lives people lead. As such they become a talking point for an ongoing dialogue, focusing on who the person is rather than simply what they have done.

Collage offers a medium where individuals are able to present and explore their lives, offering important insights into values, belief systems, their sense of humour and those hidden facets of personality that can be so easily lost or forgotten. Hopes and dreams, favourite things, love, friendship, a special place, home, achievements, belonging are all themes I have used as the starting point of collage work. Their ambivalence means that the person chooses whether they relate only to the past or whether the present and future feature in the work. Harry, for example, explored the food within the broader theme of 'my favourite things'. Whilst images of tapioca pudding reminiscent of school dinners were a strong feature, so too were items from the care home menu.

The final pieces are unique and beautiful, capturing individual personalities. This might find expression in the way the images are meticulously ordered, the colours used, or the content of the image. During one very memorable exchange George, a person with dementia staying on a respite ward, built his collage based on 'friendships' around a menagerie of pets – past and present. It spoke volumes. His daughter on seeing this laughed and said it was *'typically Dad'*.

Husbands, wives and grandchildren have also embraced this medium, possibly because it is so accessible and something people feel they can easily share. In these instances it has offered a mechanism through which family members are able to explore an evolving and sometimes fractured relationship. The final piece is an expression of a longer journey they have travelled together. This act of making can be incredibly healing and I have seen family members create their own life-story works as expressions of the relationship they have (*Things I love about you Mum*) or as a way of offering an additional perspective (*Things to know and understand about Dad*). Some carers and family members I have worked alongside have found this too difficult to do and the feelings too raw to process, whilst others have found it exceptionally helpful, a celebration of life as expressed by the following quote by a daughter:

> *This process has reminded me about the importance of the detail – those tiny facets and facts it's easy to forget. It shows you the sacrifices she made – the time she pawned her wedding ring so that we could all have a decent pair of shoes for school or when she gave up her bedroom so we had a place to live when the business fell through. It makes me feel incredibly humble.*

Whilst most collages are contained on sheets of paper or card this does not always have to be the case. Collage can overflow onto other surfaces and be used to decorate small pieces of furniture, books, or boxes. One of the most beautiful examples of life-story work I have seen was in a hospital in Derbyshire where boxes were adorned with images chosen by the person with dementia as being significant. Inside the box were six or seven objects each of which reflected something about the person; their interests, things they valued. The combined effect was to present a three-dimensional picture of that individual as well as to offer a starting point to discover more.

Tom Kitwood (1997) wrote 'in dementia the sense of identity based on having a life story to tell may eventually fade. When it does biographical knowledge about a person becomes essential if that identity is still to be held in place' (Kitwood 1997, p.56). Collage offers one medium through which it is possible to do this. Above all it represents an encounter, a tangible meeting space where much can be communicated and learned about who someone is whether this is through the materials they choose or the words that are spoken.

In the arts box

Scissors.

Pencils.

Glue.

Light card.

Mount spray.

Magazines, brochures, pictures, maps, music sheets.

Paint, paint brushes.

(Access to a photocopier).

TRY-OUTS

When you think of paper, what picture comes into mind? A4 writing paper, a sheet of A3 paper, graph paper? Let's begin with a simple activity. How many different kinds of paper can you name? Photographic paper, tissue paper, greaseproof paper, envelopes, books, wallpaper, drawing paper, handmade paper, writing paper, newspaper, crepe paper.

Take a sheet of paper and make three tears in this. The first time you do this tear it in a way to express anger, the second, in a way to express joy, the third time in such a way to express feelings of peace or relaxation. Now see how many other emotions you can inject into the tears.

Take another sheet of paper and see how many ways you can fold this. Note how the qualities of the paper change as you do this and it becomes more robust, stronger.

See if you can find a sheet of paper that reflects something about who you are. Would you be a sheet of newspaper, containing lots of facts, quite black and white in your thinking or a layer of shocking pink tissue paper? Would you be patterned or plain? What texture would you be: flexible, smooth or stiff and less pliable?

Look through magazines and newspapers and see if you can find headlines or titles of articles that sum up exactly how you feel.

Look again through a series of magazines and newspapers. This time try to find images that tell your story. This time no words are allowed. Imagine that you are sharing these images with a stranger. What do you think they would convey to that person?

14.

Further Than the Eye Can See[2]

Claire Craig

We take photographs for many reasons – fun, recreation, to document events reminding us that we were in a certain place at a certain time.

Photographs provide a tangible record, a prompt for memory, with potential to aid recall. John Berger (1992, p.192) said that *'the thrill found in a photograph comes from the onrush of memory.'* This can be very true and for this reason photographs have been used extensively with people with dementia as a prompt for reminiscence supporting communication by enabling the person to access past memories (Rentz 1995; Gibson 2004; Cappeliez *et al.* 2005)

However, place a camera in the hands of a person with dementia and we see a different picture. Here the camera becomes a tool for exploration and experimentation with a focus on the present, offering an outlet for self-expression. The person is active, in control of the process and the images produced offer a glimpse of the world through their eyes which can offer new insights and understanding.

---

2 The title of this chapter 'Further Than the Eye Can See' was inspired by the article 'Photo elicitaion and research with men' by John Oliffe and Joan Bottorff in the *Journal of Qualitive Health Research* 2007, 17, 850.

'Captured Memories' (Mitchell 2005) is an illustration of what can happen when people with dementia are supported to take their own photographs. The project, facilitated by Rosas Mitchell invited individuals attending a drop-in centre to participate in a series of community outings and to create their own personal records of the experience using disposable cameras. The accounts shared by people taking part are remarkable in terms of the breadth of opportunities the experience provided. One person for instance used the photographs as a concrete reminder of what occurred. Rosas describes how:

> 'at first his memory of the sequence of events held more truth for him than the numbers on the back of the photographs. He used the latter to aid his memory and it became like a mini detective story. Yes, he must have gone back for that second cup of coffee!!' (Mitchell 2005, p.19).

The process was powerful in reinforcing a sense of self and building esteem. Participants expressed pleasure in the work produced: 'I have never taken such a good photograph'; 'I was very doubtful at first but I am very pleased with the results' and in the relationships they formed, 'I like to detect the people in the photos'; 'I like to see myself smiling.'

Some participants spoke through the images. 'You get what you take so you have to make sure that you take what you want' was one telling comment, the photograph acting as a visual metaphor.

It is this quality of the photograph to act as a visual metaphor and offer a glimpse of the inner landscape that makes it an ideal medium for expressive work for people with dementia. The work of James McKillop is a powerful testament to this. James became an accomplished artist following a diagnosis of dementia. His published book of photographs *Opening Shutters Opening Minds* is striking both in terms of the technical accuracy of the images and their emotive qualities – an extension of his inner landscape. The images are subtle, powerful (an example of one of his colour photographs can be found in the central colour section of this book). Other people with dementia have used photography to express their experience more directly. This is evident in the work of William Utermohlen (www.williamutermohlen.org) who used the camera and paint to visually chronicle his experience. His 'self-portraits' speak for themselves, powerful visual statements of the experience of living with dementia, requiring no verbal narrative.

This expressive quality of photographs makes the medium particularly accessible for individuals who struggle with verbal communication. Also photography doesn't carry the same loaded issues of other visual art forms in terms of 'good art' or 'bad art' and does not require the same investment of time or energy. Many people have owned a camera at some point in their lives and have either taken photographs of others or had their photograph taken so it is a familiar medium. As such photography can be developed into a valued leisure pursuit and shared with others. The camera also offers the person a sense of control. Some of the clearest illustrations of this are the video-portraits of people with dementia created by Sitar Rose. She works alongside individuals in such a way that they direct the film-making process, sometimes taking hold of the video camera, sometimes telling Sitar what to film. The end pieces are beautiful representations of a shared process that has taken place and the relationship that has developed through this.

Within photography, the building of relationship can occur at so many different points in the process, whether this is through the act of taking a picture or in the sharing of the image. When John Berger said:

'The thrill found in a photograph comes from the onrush of memory.'
he later added:

This is obvious when it's a picture of something we once knew. That house we lived in. Mother, when young. But in another sense, we once knew everything we recognise in any photo. That's grass growing. Tiles on a roof get wet like that, don't they? Here is one of the seven ways in which bosses smile…memory is a strange faculty. The sharper and more isolated the stimulus memory receives, the more it remembers. (Berger 1992, p.192–93)

Images are not neutral objects but loaded with emotion. When a person with dementia takes and shares an image or a piece of video footage with you they are inviting you to step into their world, surrendering important clues about their values, friendships, key life events, paths they have trodden. The process of sharing this story can be relationship forming in a way that goes beyond a simple conversation. It is necessary to remember that you will also bring to the image a set of experiences that will shape your response. We must be sensitive to and mindful of the power of this process. I have witnessed first hand the tensions that can arise when the person with dementia is using the photograph as a medium through which to share powerful emotions and a family member is reading the image as a factual account, part of their history.

My starting point then is always to build an understanding of what photographs mean to a person. When I work alongside individuals I like to begin the process of introducing the person to the medium by sharing an old shoe box full of random photographs collected over the years. I sit by the person and we look through the pictures together. This simple process leads to natural conversations about image making. Here I discover much about the person. For instance, who the main photographer was in the family, whether this is an activity the person has enjoyed, something about the types of subjects they photograph (landscapes, portraits) and even where and how photographs are stored (ordered in albums or lose in shoe boxes and carrier bags). Gradually I can begin to understand where image making fits in the context of the person's life, their likes and dislikes and a bit about who they are.

In a subsequent session I like to invite the person to choose one or two photographs and to give each one a title or a name. This helps to move away from only ever seeing a photograph as a factual record and offers an opportunity for self-expression, a way to exercise the imagination. Elaborate stories can flow from the simplest of photographs as the following responses by people with dementia to the following image, show:

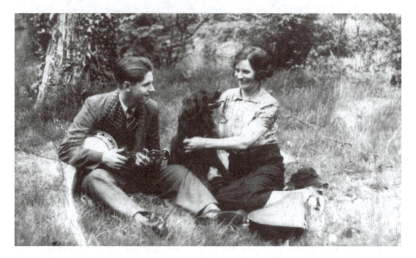

'The title is sunlight serenade'.

'It is called "only eyes for you".' He thinks she is hopelessly in love with him (laughs) but what he doesn't realise is that she is looking at the dog!!

'A secret encounter': I don't think they are married by the way they are sitting. She has put the dog in the middle as a sort of chaperone.

Once I feel that I am developing an understanding as to the person's relationship with images and image making we then engage in the photographic process. On one level photography groups where people with dementia are invited to take photographs will flourish with little input from the facilitator. However, too much choice and no direction can sometimes be disabling and it can therefore be helpful to offer people structures and themes for image making including ways of using the photographs once they have been taken. Photography around a theme can be particularly useful here. For instance you may use this as an opportunity to find out more about the person, using the image-making process to reinforce identity; 'my favourite things'; 'a special place'; 'food, glorious food'; 'self-portrait' are examples of themes you might use.

You may choose to focus the process around a particular activity. For instance 'taking a camera for a walk' where individuals choose a place or a route they would like to go and use this as a springboard for taking photographs also works particularly well. Even within this the person or group may choose to select particular themes to photograph: magic moments, unusual views, colour, texture, are all examples of this. When you are out on the walk you are well advised to remember Alfred Wainwright's famous saying 'always stop and look'. This will help to reduce the possibility of trips and slips.

Once the photographs have been developed they can offer opportunities for discussion, starting points for further creative ventures including as a stimulus for creative writing and poetry. 'Focusing on the Person', a resource available from Stirling Dementia Services Development Centre offers a number of ways of using images creatively (Craig 2005).

Up to this point I have said something about the why and what of photography. Now I turn to the how. Personally I find that using my own camera and taking pictures alongside the person in a session feels very natural and provides plenty of scope for discussion, for sharing skills and models the process. This can help individuals who struggle to sequence the process or lack confidence in using a camera. It also means that photography becomes a shared activity with the person as opposed to something you are just observing. It is worth saying something about equipment here. Often people feel most comfortable using their own camera, one they are familiar with. I also bring to sessions throw-away and inexpensive digital cameras. In my experience people have found the digital camera easier to use; in part this is because of the clear display panel, the size of the shutter release and also the speed with which images can be printed. Throw-away cameras can present more challenges for some older people who struggle with the winding mechanism because of physical problems such as arthritis.

Over time I have also discovered that it is not necessary for a person to always physically take the photograph. Individuals unable to do this can gain just as much through the process of talking about, planning and putting together a composition. A cardboard frame can emulate the viewfinder to assist in this activity.

The focus here is on shared relationship and the opportunity for the person to highlight what is important. As John Eno-Daynes reflects in his work with individuals with dementia:

People demonstrated real concern and awareness about composition, colour, subject…I was amazed by the subtlety of their communication and how much was evident in terms of creativity and desire for self-expression. (Eno-Daynes 2000, p.3)

Photographs and film then represent meeting places, can provide scaffolds for conversation acting as visual prompts, providing an outlet for self-expression and helping us to see the world through someone else's eyes. The process is powerful; the visual and visible nature of images can be exposing and you will need to help your participants to find their own comfort zone when exploring images, remembering that at all times the image belongs to the person and as such they are in complete control as to how this should be used and who should view it.

However, offering a person with dementia the opportunity to take their own photographs is the act of inviting that individual to seek out new experiences, new memories, with the potential to build deeper relationships and discover new worlds that extend further than the eye can see.

TRY-OUTS

Look through your album at home and find a picture that best sums up who you are… Now imagine that you are trying to impress someone. What picture would you choose now? How does this differ from the first one?

Building on this theme of a self-portrait take your camera and try and build up a visual picture about who you are, find images that captures what motivates you, what angers you, what you dream about, your hopes, your wishes.

Set these out in front of you. Looking at the pictures, does anything surprise you? How did it feel to do this activity?

Are there any pictures you would feel uncomfortable sharing with others? How might it feel to be asked to share these?

Look through a series of newspapers and magazines. See if you can find an image that captures something of the exact opposite of who you are. For example, if you are very neat and tidy, find a picture of chaos. When you have found this image, stick it to your fridge and revisit it from time to time. What do you learn about yourself through that image? What might this tell you?

15.

Putting the IT into Creativity

Exploring the Creative Potential of Technology

Claire Craig

We live in a world surrounded by technology: computers, palm-tops and mobile phones permeate much of what we do. We can sometimes associate such gadgets with function and functionality rather than as tools for leisure and recreation. You can see this emphasis in relation to people with dementia where much energy has been devoted over the last few years to the development of electronic way-finding devices, prompts to help memory and devices to increase safety by automatically turning off gas or water taps.

Yet technology also offers tremendous opportunities for engagement, play, exploration and self-expression. If you are in any doubt just pause for a moment and think about what technology offers in the context of your own life whether it is listening to music, taking photographs using a digital camera, playing computer games or keeping in touch with family and friends through e-mail. These devices hold much creative potential for people with dementia. A person I was working with recently declared the computer to be '*a window into another world*' and another person as a '*new adventure*'.

So what does this technology look like? Over the last few years a number of specialist products have emerged that are able to bring together digital music, reminiscence, touch screens and art (Topo *et al.* 2004). However, our emphasis here is on using everyday technology, those pieces of equipment that are familiar, affordable, accessible and can be shared with families and friends. Examples of such technologies would include equipment that you would find in most homes or care environments – mobile telephones, computers, cameras, video and tape recorders. The biggest advantage of this approach is that it helps to prevent the technology from becoming the most important element of the interaction. What we mean here is that sometimes when a new 'all-singing, all-dancing' product comes onto the market it is easy for the product to become the focus rather than the person. Technology is simply a tool, the equivalent of a paintbrush in art, a pen in poetry – a medium through which to express creativity.

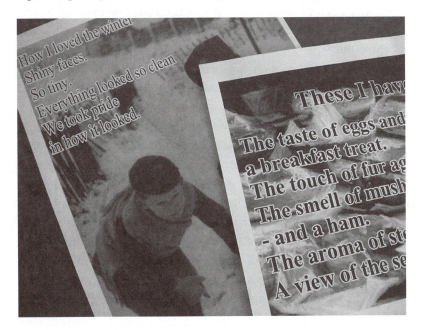

The computer offers a way of presenting creative work

At its simplest level technology offers a stimulus for creativity. Jack, the person declaring the computer as *'a window to another world'* was a keen artist and had just been on a tour of the Louvre in Paris via the Internet from the comfort of his room. He recalled in marvellous detail a previous visit, taking the lead in describing various pictures and taking inspiration from this by movingly creating his 'Mona Louisa' in pastels in memory of his wife. On-line galleries, exhibitions, music and maps can form creative activities in their own right or act as stimuli for poetry, writing, visual art, drama or music composition. As a facilitator I regularly tap into Internet sites dedicated to arts activities. Artz for Alzheimers, Timeslips and Dementiapositive (these websites are fully referenced at the end of the book) are just three examples of sites that provide creative inspiration, instructions, ideas and materials for sessions.

Technology is also a vehicle for creativity, take for example a dictaphone or tape recorder. This has formed the means for collecting, generating sounds, words and music to illustrate visual images, as a mechanism to build verbal montages or compose original music, a way to record anthologies of poetry and as a tool for storytelling. 'Pass it on' is an example of a collective storytelling project. A person began the story with a single sentence and the tape recorder was then passed to someone else in the care home. They listened to this contribution and then added another sentence and so on. The project generated huge momentum and the tape recorder was taken home by family members, carers and friends, who all contributed something to the tale. The end result was a marvellous testimony to the individuals who took part, their sense of fun and inventiveness and to the creative process itself. It also offered a powerful mechanism for building community.

These techniques work just as well with other technological media. For instance blogs and wikis can form a similar vehicle and offer the opportunity to involve family members. One relative said of the experience:

> *Although I've lived in the States for the last two years, I don't think that I've ever felt quite so close to Mum. No expectations, no pressures and a sense that throughout it all we were connected, doing it together.*

When different technologies are combined, the results can be dramatic. I have been involved in an intergenerational project called Arthouse: growing up and growing old in care, working alongside people with dementia living in care homes and looked-after children in residential care. The work has included the use of digital photography and computers to create three-dimensional portraits of who people are. In another project, 'Now and Then' participants have created compilations of 'my life as music', built up digital scrapbooks combining words and photographs and used free computer packages to integrate still images with audio accounts to create powerful digital narratives that are played as short films. One person with dementia said of her work, *'It's something to help you find your way back'* and a staff member reflected, *'The work really has reminded me that people have exceptional talents in spite of dementia. It's nice to see this.'*

Technology can be a means through which to present and share creative works. The Internet, social networking, on-line galleries all offer the opportunity for people living with dementia to showcase their art, poetry, film and music. Technology provides a platform to a worldwide audience and an opportunity for individuals to be celebrated as artists, challenging some of the preconceptions and stigma that exists in relation to what a diagnosis of dementia means. It also creates a community where individuals can offer support and encouragement and inspire others by sharing their work and experiences. Leah, a person with dementia has used her blog, a type of on-line journal, to display examples of her poetry and photography. Here are just two extracts from the blog…

I have taken up photography… it seems to be one of a few things I am still pretty good at doing. This is our baby robin on his/her first day out of the nest… I love the little pin feathers saying, 'I'm not quite finished yet…' just like me. I am not finished yet either, though I have recently been diagnosed with early onset dementia.

These poems especially help me to deal with my situation today. It helps me to put into perspective where I am, who I am, what I am. Reading these poems helps me to define the strengths I do have. The promise. It allows me to put behind me those unkind, unthinking people who do not understand dementia... and me. (www. healthcentral.com)

This reflective quality should not be overlooked. Perhaps one of the little spoken strengths of technology is that it offers distance. Possibly because it presents the work in a slightly different way or at least allows it to be viewed as such. One of the most moving examples of this was a session I was privy to where a group of individuals were photographed (with their consent) engaging in a group painting activity. The images from the digital camera were downloaded into a presentation package and projected onto a screen with accompanying words and music. The work was stunning. Rather than comprising a series of separate photographs, the images that unfolded were a dance, a beautiful work of art and a testament to the relationship and bonds between group members.

Where pieces of art, writing and textiles are photographed using a digital camera, these can be stored for posterity on the computer, viewed as collections providing a sense of coherence and continuity, and as the focus for discussion and a reminder of what someone has achieved. Technology can support a more intimate sharing or creation of these works. For instance, mobile telephones and digital picture frames offer a means through which to display photographs, or they can act as a medium to assemble three-dimensional life stories, including images and recorded narratives.

More recently a range of affordable computers with highly accessible touch screens have come onto the market, the size of a book which make it possible to sit alongside the person, navigating between pages, and zooming in on detail, all through touch.

It is perhaps unsurprising then that these technological media can operate as meeting places between different generations. A person recently told me:

No-one and I mean no-one in my family is artistic – that's what makes the computer so perfect for Dad. He can print things out. No mistakes. My grandson showed him Paintbrush – a kind of arts package. Well if you could have seen them both. It was amazing.

The family went on to create a history of the family using a simple presentation package transforming reminiscence into a treasured heirloom.

Another carer on seeing how it was possible to embed words in a photograph using a simple word processing package said:

> *I'd not thought much about using the computer like but I'm just thinking of one person who loves to write poetry. She would love to learn how to do this and the end results would be brilliant. It really has got me thinking and it is so simple.*

Clearly there are things to be aware of. The cost of the technology for one, although for a small amount of money invested it is possible to create multiple opportunities for individuals, their families and friends. There are also ethical questions to consider, particularly if a person wants to share their work with a broader audience through the Internet. However, by the same token people at an early point in their dementia journey have spoken about how they have appreciated the anonymity of being able to post things onto the Internet without being judged or questioned or everything being attributed to dementia.

People with dementia will approach technology with varying levels of confidence and skill. Generalisations can often be made in terms of what people can and cannot achieve. Yet research has shown that:

> *people with dementia can engage in computer work at many different levels... the common misconception is that people with dementia cannot learn new skills or be able to benefit from being involved in interacting with computers which is untrue.* (Social Care Institute for Excellence: Good Practice Example 01)

Where a person is less confident emphasis can be placed on offering support and 'sharing technology together'.

When I first began working as an occupational therapist she was told, *'The computer is a work-tool, not a playground.'* With this attitude technology can sometimes be confined to the realm of report writing and word processing. However, the scope of this medium in relation to creativity should not be underestimated. If you are unsure you only need to listen to the voice of people with dementia who are discovering what it holds and encouraging others to do the same. In the words of Leah, a person with dementia:

I have just recently bought a computer program which will allow me to do digital scrapbooking. This is a wonderful invention for people such as myself who have a short-term memory problems. This program allows me to change backgrounds until I find one I like. Then I can arrange pictures and embellish them with corners, flowers, flourishes, etc. I can journal anywhere on the page I wish. With all the choices I have, my mind is exercised to its max. I strongly recommend early onset dementia people to get out and take pictures and put them onto some type of digital scrapbook. Your mind will be used through making endless choices and critiquing your work as you go. And, in the end, you will have something to show others and to be proud of. (www.healthcentral.com)

TRY-OUTS

Think about your own interests and home; list all the ways you use technology to engage in creative and leisure activities. Useful starting points might include: listening to music, watching films, playing games, digital picture frames.

If you have access to a computer and the Internet see how many creative activities you can engage in from the comfort of your front room. For instance you might decide to go for a walk in the park, view an exhibition at an art gallery, wander around a museum, find or compose a poem.

Share a piece of technology with someone you are working with. Invite the person to describe some of the technologies of 'their day'.

16.

Space and Place

The Environment and Creativity

Claire Craig

Have you ever looked out over a landscape or gazed at a sunset and felt so overwhelmed by its beauty that momentarily it has taken your breath away? Can you recall a time when you have visited an exhibition or attended a theatrical production and have been so transfixed that you have momentarily been transported somewhere else? Let's try an opposite tack. How about places you have found so oppressive that you just wanted to leave: rooms with no windows, dreary carpets, oppressive noise, suffocating heat, not enough air? We can all identify places like this.

We often think about the environment in relation to its physical dimensions rather than our emotional response, the way it makes us feel and act. At its best the space we inhabit has the potential to inspire and feed our spirit, foster creativity and promote feelings of wellbeing. A recent systematic review of the arts for health literature looking how visual art and design impacted on the wellbeing of people living and working in healthcare settings concluded that design and decoration can promote wellbeing and improve physical and psychological functioning (Ulrich 1992 in Staricoff 2004) The findings of this review are not new. As early as 1859 Florence Nightingale (Notes on Nursing) observed:

> *The effect of beautiful objects, of variety of objects and especially of brilliance of colour is hardly at all appreciated... I have seen in fevers the most acute suffering produced from the patient not being able to see out of a window and the knots in the wood being the only view. I shall never forget the rapture of fever patients over a bunch of bright coloured flowers. Little as we know about the way in which we are affected by form, by colour, and light, we do know this, that they have an actual physical effect. Variety of form and brilliancy of colour in the objects presented to patients are actual means of recovery.* (Nightingale, 1859 quoted in Department of Health 2007 p.2)

There is strong evidence to show how art and architecture help people with dementia to be orientated within their environment (Passini *et al.* 1995) and can also reduce anxiety and increase wellbeing (Lovell *et al.* 1995; Cooper and Barnes 1995; Day *et al.* 2000; Teresi *et al.* 2000; Haq and Zimring 2003). Indeed, the arts in their broader sense offer a valuable source of stimulation, (Miles 1994; Cooper *et al.* 1995) promoting discussion, offering a focus for communication and creating an ambience whether this is through the images hanging on the walls or music playing in the background (Craig 2002). For people at a more advanced point in their journey through dementia, finding ways to create a textured environment is particularly important. Ways to do this include tactile blankets, wall-hangings and making nice materials available for people to interact with (bowls of felt balls, silk scarves).

Clearly then a precedent exists to support the inclusion of artworks in hospitals and care settings. This does not have to be expensive. By far the most effective way to do this is to invite people with dementia to exhibit some of the art, poetry, photographs and sculpture they have created. In this way individuals are able to put their mark on the places in which they live and the environment becomes an extension of self and a reinforcement of identity. One particularly vivid memory was whilst I was working as an occupational therapist. I had a follow-up visit to see Maria, a person with dementia who had recently been discharged from the hospital to a care environment. She had little verbal speech and on arrival took my hand and led me to her room where a painting she had created during an arts session on the ward had been framed and hung. She was thrilled with this and staff in the home described how this had prompted them to purchase a small pad of watercolour paper and some paints. The painting had helped staff to see beyond the label of dementia and understand something about who she was. In framing and celebrating her work, the staff and other residents were also celebrating something of her. Other individuals have indicated that this fulfils a more basic function helping the person to recognise their room and avoid the feeling voiced by one person who said, *'I never quite know whose bed I sleep in, you know, you can never tell one from another.'*

Other ways of introducing art into the environment include accessing art loans from local libraries, offering exhibition space to local art colleges and framing prints, postcards or even recycled calendars. The key throughout all of this is to ensure that individuals living in the environment have the opportunity to choose the art that is used, since a masterpiece to one person could be a monstrosity to another.

There is another dimension to consider here in that creativity does not occur in a vacuum. It happens in a context within a broader physical, social and cultural environment. At its best this environment can inspire, nurture and provide a vehicle through which creativity can be expressed. At worst the physical setting, the attitudes of people and the broader culture can extinguish any creative sparks that have been ignited. We will first look at how the environment can inspire creativity.

Painting, drawing, photography, poetry can all be inspired by the setting in which they are created. You need only think of Wordsworth's Daffodils, Monet's Water Lilies or Van Gogh's Sunflowers to recognise the relationship between the physical environment and the creative process. Outdoor spaces can be particularly valuable in relation to this, providing a stimulus for the creative act. Engaging in creative activities outdoors whether it is painting a scene, seeking inspiration for poetry or photography on a walk offers a completely different feel to the process. For one thing there is a greater sense of freedom as you are less constrained in terms of worrying about spilling materials or in making a mess. For another, the outdoors offers a far greater sensory experience, the aromas of plants and shrubs, textures, shadows and reflections. The quality of the work produced is therefore much richer. If working outdoors isn't possible, bring elements of the outdoors in. Found objects, stones, flowers can all be used as springboards to creative work. Some plants, for example, can be woven into textiles or be incorporated into paintings or collage.

Nature also has its own creative rhythm you may tap into. I have personally found linking arts-based activities to this rhythm to be particularly effective. Christmas wreaths, outdoor carol singing around a Christmas tree, Easter egg hunts, dancing and picnics have all offered a broader context for creativity and a way to build closer links with the community. There is a lovely example of this in a community near where I live where the Chinese population of one district invite people living in a nearby care home to share in their festivities and take part in the 'festival of light' releasing hundreds of Chinese paper lanterns, lovingly made by residents, into the evening sky.

In environments where space is so often at a premium, it is nice to use outdoor spaces to display and 'frame' pieces of art that have been created offering an outdoor gallery which other residents and carers can enjoy. Naturally some materials lend themselves more easily to surviving the outdoor elements: ceramics, mosaics, and wooden structures do very well and are made for outside. However, with a little imagination it is possible to introduce other art-forms into these spaces. For example, poetry can be written or painted on stones. When varnished these pieces can add a wonderful touch and form the basis of poetry walks and storytelling. Photographs and pieces of art can also be protected from the elements when they are displayed in sealed jars or bottles. Outside spaces can offer a perfect backdrop for performances including storytelling, poetry events and evening concerts (inviting local bands or choirs to perform).

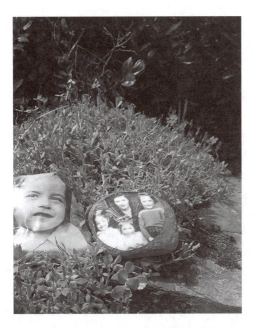

The outdoors can offer a perfect backdrop for displaying pieces of artwork

Whether the indoors or outdoors is used to inspire creativity, some practical considerations exist including the availability of chairs and surfaces to rest on and if spending time outdoors, places to sit in shaded areas away from the blistering effects of the sun. If what I have described fosters and promotes creativity, there are a number of factors that have the opposite effect and stem or at worst extinguish the creative flow. These include fixed and inflexible routines, lack of access to outside space, dimly lit environments (studies by Hughes and Neer 1981 have shown that by the age of 60 there is a 66 per cent reduction of light reaching the retina), televisions playing continuously in corners of rooms and loud music. In fact continuous background noise has been found to be one of the most disabling features of environments for people with dementia who may be struggling to concentrate and process information (Sloane *et al.* 1998).

Equally as inhibiting are some attitudes where people with dementia are seen as 'children' or infantalised, or the assumption is made that the person with dementia does not communicate, cannot feel or engage in creativity and as a consequence of this is denied the opportunity to participate. Tom Kitwood (1997) described such attitudes as part of the malignant social psychology that can sometimes pervade the environments where people with dementia live. Often not the result of malicious intent, such attitudes still have the potential to devalue, disable and dehumanise the person. Significantly Tom Kitwood (1997) also recognised the potential of creativity to counter this and affirm personhood and empower the individual.

Creativity happens in a context. Within this context it has the potential to shape the environments where people with dementia live, promoting feelings of wellbeing, providing the opportunity to promote identity and foster personhood. However, just as the wider environment can inspire creativity, by the same token it can also inhibit the creative process. In any creative approach it is therefore an area in which we need to be particularly mindful.

TRY-OUTS

- Spend a few moments thinking of or describing your favourite view or landscape. Invite friends and family members to do the same.

- Our view of outdoor space changes as time passes. How have you used space at different periods of your life?

- Plan a design of your ideal outdoor space.

- Turn a walk into an adventure, a prayer or a meditation.

- Imagine for one moment that you have been told that you are not allowed to go outside ever again. How does this feel? What do you think you would miss the most?

17.

Taking It All In

Audience Enjoyment

John Killick

So far all our short chapters describing artforms have been about taking part. This one is a compendium of ways in which people with dementia can experience appreciation either individually or as part of a group. In the world beyond dementia there are many more people who go to concerts than play instruments; who go to galleries than paint pictures; who read books than write them. It could be that with people with the condition, because of the desperate need for activity, we may need to attempt to change this equation. Nevertheless there will be many people who will enjoy works made by others. Using the senses and the imagination on already existing artefacts is itself a creative process and can lead to heightened awareness and an increased sense of wellbeing. What follow are a number of examples of this in practice.

Going to the pictures

I have run video and photography appreciation sessions which I call 'Going to the Pictures', because I want the concept to be familiar and unthreatening. In each case I have managed to secure a room which could be blacked out so that the environment of a cinema could be simulated. I have had the assistance of excellent video and DVD equipment and a large screen TV so that high quality vision and sound was assured. Five or six individuals participated at a time.

Each of the one-hour sessions followed the same pattern: two video extracts followed by discussion (with appropriate action replays to bring out details) and two segments looking at photographs, one of which involved single large reproductions being passed round the group for comments, and the other a different photograph for each member of the group before it was passed round. All the pictures were gleaned from newspapers and magazines and were sturdy, mounted on card and laminated. The photography and video segments were alternated for the sake of variety.

I had already decided that this was not to be a reminiscence project. I wanted to see how people reacted to materials that were unfamiliar. Therefore, none of the photographs were of local scenes or people, or if they were reproductions of paintings they would not be of the most popular works, and none of the video extracts came from films which the participants were likely to know. Examples of videos used were the Jacques Tati films *Jour de Fete* and *Mon Oncle*, the film *Saltimbanco* from *Cirque Du Soleil*, experimental shorts by the Canadian filmmaker Norman McLaren, and the BBC nature film *Deep Blue*.

Almost without exception group members settled down to the activity within minutes, and this usually included people who found difficulty in concentrating. Sometimes in the discussions people took off into remarkable flights of fancy: one lady said, '*Something in that film just started me off.*' At one point I showed a collage made by Ray Maloney, a man with dementia, entitled *Blues in the Night*. One participant commented, '*I know exactly how he feels. I fell off a bridge and injured my head. It affected my memory badly, but it is gradually returning. It is helped by times like this.*'

I have learned that it doesn't much matter what visual material you choose to present so long as it is bold and clear. A couple of the video extracts used proved too complex for people to unravel. And the photographs mustn't be too ambiguous. The fact that none of the subjects was familiar did not seem to be of consequence. Anyone who wished to reminisce was free to do so: one lady even related a picture of an elephant in India to her childhood park in Edinburgh!

On a much larger scale, the Artz for Alzheimers scheme in the USA takes large numbers of seniors to the cinema for reminiscence sessions. One such event occurred in Boston in Spring 2010; it was one of four visits. About 200 participants gathered in the Coolidge Corner Theatre for extracts from old movies, such as *Oklahoma*, *Casablanca* and *The Wizard of Oz*, popcorn and soda provided.

In between the clips the audience was quizzed by a pair of interlocutors. One of the questioners introduced the extracts, giving in turn information about each and setting the scene emotionally for what was to follow. The other exercised a role after each clip by attempting to elicit reactions from members of the audience by asking questions like 'What feelings does that evoke in you?' and to relate it in general terms to events in people's lives like 'Did anything like that happen to you?' There was never any difficulty in obtaining responses from a deeply involved group of people. The answers received from such queries were amazingly detailed and often personally revealing. Although only a small number of people could speak out, many others became involved by voicing assent or chorusing disagreement. The sense of a shared experience was palpable, and an observer commented on the extent of knowledge displayed and the quality of the insights shared.

Going to the gallery

The movement to bring people with dementia to works of art is growing apace worldwide. There is no reason why people who enjoyed visiting galleries prior to dementia should not continue to do so, and it is also an activity which could develop as a new-found enthusiasm (Killick 2008b).

The Hearthstone Foundation in America was established in 1992 by John Zeisel. One arm of the organisation consists of a number of assisted living care homes in New York City and State, and Massachusetts. Another is the Museums Partnership programme. This was piloted at the Museum of Modern Art in New York. Members of staff were trained to run sessions looking at paintings with groups of people with dementia. The museum arranged the programme on the day it was closed so as to avoid distraction, and the visiting group gathered before a Van Gogh, Matisse or Monet and was led in a discussion.

The New York Times carried an article with a lively description of one of these sessions. Oliver Sacks, the neurologist, commented on the process:

> Certainly it's not just a visual experience – it's an emotional one. In an informal way I have often seen quite demented patients recognise and respond vividly to paintings and delight in painting at a time when they are scarcely responsive to words and disoriented out of it. I think that recognition of visual art can be very deep.

The Museums Partnership Programme now includes a variety of institutions in a number of countries, including France, Spain and Britain. At the National Gallery of Australia, where a pilot project was carried out, participants were commenting on a painting by Russell Drysdale entitled 'A Sunday Walk' which showed a father and two children holding hands on a street where all the windows were painted black. The discussion was about the buildings and what Drysdale meant by the way he had painted them. One person said, 'The windows were dirty and this morning I had my windows cleaned.' The accompanying caregiver was astonished by the comment because that morning the cleaning crew had arrived as they were leaving for the museum. Her short-term memory cued by the painting was clearly intact.

It is just as important for people with dementia to encounter works of art by others with the condition as it is to create them:

the one activity feeds off the other in terms of stimulus and the engendering of a sense of possibility and achievement. The Artz project accomplishes this as well. Exhibitions of artworks produced are mounted and toured. One person who went to see such an exhibition commented:

> *I was moved by the feelings that washed over me. I could feel the artists' energies coming off the pieces. They are in there!!! and how wonderfull (sic) to communicate in this way – no misunderstandings – right here now, their feelings.*

Enjoying music

If there are such things as platitudes in the subject of communication with people with dementia, that of the response to music of individuals and groups whatever their level of difficulty is one. There are now so many accounts of persons who appear to be locked into their own private worlds, hardly responding to any stimulus provided and apparently only intermittently, if at all, appearing to recognise their loved ones, yet moving fingers and/ or toes, or smiling, or making gestures of recognition when familiar music is played, that we can take this phenomenon as a given. We want to reinforce the message that non-verbal language, and its powerful emotional appeal, must be a first port-of call in any artistic initiative involving a possible 'awakening' of anyone considered difficult to reach.

We will allow ourselves one example only, and this is taken from a film entitled *Black Daisies for the Bride* devised by the poet Tony Harrison for the BBC in 1990, and filmed in the long-stay ward of a hospital in Leeds. There is a particularly telling episode where a woman whom we have seen earlier in the film speaking to no-one, but engaged in dusting the ledges in a lounge, is suddenly confronted by an entertainer, Richard Muttonchops, who is singing and playing a guitar. He addresses his music specifically to her, and begins singing 'Oh You Beautiful Doll'. At first she has her back to him, but she quickly turns, her eyes lighting up. She is soon fully engaged, dancing and singing along with him;

she makes up her own words to the tune. Though she is probably in her 70s or 80s, the years fall away before our eyes, and she is a young woman again responding ardently to the advances of a lover. The words and music, whether by accident or design, are perfectly suited to the occasion.

The organisation in the UK which has most experience of providing music for people with dementia is 'Music for Life'. It is based in London, and was founded by Linda Rose in 1993. It uses professional musicians, and offers them special training for the work. Care staff are also encouraged to become involved and are offered special training. Here is a description of the process of a session:

> *Musicians interact with participants using a variety of instruments. This enables people who may be isolated and disempowered, as a result of losses associated with the later stages of Alzheimer's and other forms of dementia, to explore, enjoy, discover, reminisce, and communicate in new ways, identifying and building on areas still intact.* (Rose 2008, p.21)

Linda Rose and Stephanie Schlingensiepen (2010) outline their attempt to build confidence and provide stimulus in a manner which they term 'safe unpredictability'. The familiar and the new are brought into a fruitful equilibrium. They state:

> *Increasingly during the sessions we are privileged to participate in something beyond the ordinary, where some deep if momentary link has occurred between people in the group. Annie, for example, with the expressiveness of her eyes and only minimal hand-movements, inspired a deeply moving improvisation supported by the silent, almost tangible focus of the rest of the group. These are moments to be recognised and cherished – when something beyond words or music has been at work and something essentially human and life-enhancing has been touched.* (Rose 2008, p.21)

In a later, and most insightful article, Linda Rose (2010), and staff from the Jewish Care Homes where much of their pioneering work has been carried out, tell how projects have awakened and fostered the creativity of staff as well as residents, so much so that, through the reflective practice involved, they have come to be regarded as a model for staff development.

Enjoying poetry

Here are some comments by individuals with dementia:

This is good. The more you hear of it the more you pick up that different thing that's needed.

It moves you, I mean, it hits you inside where it meets you and means something.

Thank you. I had a wonderful time. I love this every week. It's good to be here.

I like the way it flows together. The words flow into one another, but they're all separate somehow and not the same.

They are special moments, especially if you haven't read for weeks, and then you read this here and it touches you and you realise how much you have been longing for it really. I love poetry.

The last quote provides the clue to the activity all five persons are taking part in: the shared reading of poems in a group. 'Get Into Reading' is an outreach project run by the Reader Organization in Merseyside, which has been growing over a number of years (Killick 2008a). The moving force is Jane Davis, who was editor of *The Reader* magazine until this major initiative demanded all her attention.

The project worker from the outset has been Katie Peters. She developed the activity very much on a trial-and-error basis. When she began she was unsure of what would work with the client group. She tried prose, both fiction and non-fiction, but people had difficulty with remembering plot-lines. Wordsworth's 'The Daffodils' provided her with her first success, and she soon found other classic poems that many remembered from their schooldays (Masefield's 'Sea Fever' and Burns's 'My Love is Like a Red Red Rose', for instance). She has discovered, however, that some texts that are unfamiliar to everyone also make a strong impact. The very strangeness of the language, she suggests, may encourage people to seek out meaning.

Each group is usually made up of about eight participants, including family carers and a staff member as well as people with dementia. A range of communication difficulties is accommodated as Katie finds that those with greater fluency encourage those who have various barriers to expressing themselves.

The poems are chosen carefully as a mix of the familiar and the new, and large-print copies are provided for everyone. Katie reads each one aloud, and others are encouraged to join in. The discussions are free and frank, taking in meanings and feelings.

Katie adopts the same style and uses the same material when she is working one-to-one. These sessions are really a way of allowing those with dementia who would otherwise be unable or unwilling to attend groups the opportunity to participate. Some may be bed-bound, others may not react well to the presence of other residents. She offers them a pleasurable activity in surroundings in which they feel comfortable and secure.

Is there something about poetry that gives it a special appeal to people with dementia? Katie thinks so:

There is definitely something about the rhythm and rhyme of poetry that encourages people. I have seen people tapping on the table in time with the rhythm, and often those who cannot read along like to 'join in' in this way by feeling part of the thing. We found early on that prose did not hold people's attention, but the poetry received a completely different reaction, with people leaning forward in their chairs and wanting to join in. (p.29)

I do believe that there is more to it than the rhyme and rhythm though. I have observed that much of the communication in the care home is hurried and confused. It is hard for residents to engage well with staff or with other residents, lost as they are in their own world and way of thinking. When you read a poem through slowly the rhythm of it actually slows you down. It gives people the opportunity to pause for a moment, to come away from the chaos and to stay with one line or one word, and to really think about the meaning behind it. Each word is chosen so carefully and precisely in poetry that meaning is very important. Often people repeat a line or phrase that they liked and we take that as a starting-point. It is wonderful to see people communicating well over the poems, using them as a shared point of focus. We can read a poem through a few times too and give it time to settle in and resonate. (p.29)

TRY-OUTS

What has been the most moving/enjoyable film/exhibition/play/concert you have seen? What made it so?

Are there any plays/exhibitions/concerts/galleries that you always wanted to go to but didn't have the chance? If you could go to just one play what would that be?

Design your perfect day/evening out. Where would you go, what would you see?

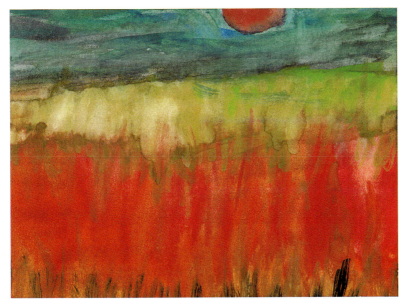

'Hot Summer' by Burt (Albert) Reynolds. Following his diagnosis Burt discovered a love for landscape painting.

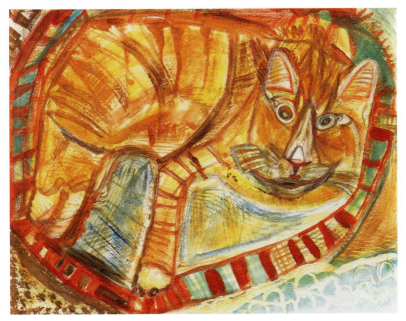

'Harry the Handsome Cat' by David Whitcombe. David created this work during his involvement in an Alzheimer Society-funded art group in Shrewsbury run by Elisha Maran-Barnell.

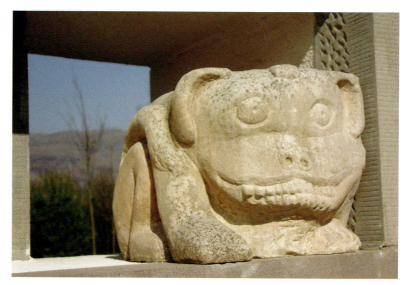

'Guard Dog' by Christophe Grillet. Christophe took up sculpture following his diagnosis of dementia and this is just one of a number of pieces he has created.

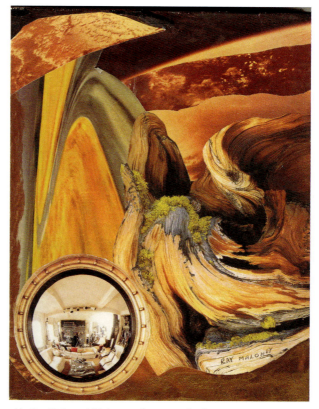

'Safe Haven' by Ray Maloney. This is one of a series of collages created by Ray. He makes the following comment about the medium, 'I liked the idea that I could pick up a collage and work on it it. It didn't matter that I couldn't remember where I left off.'

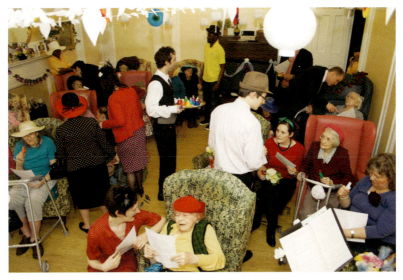

Ladder to the Moon is a London-based theatre company that functions in care settings.

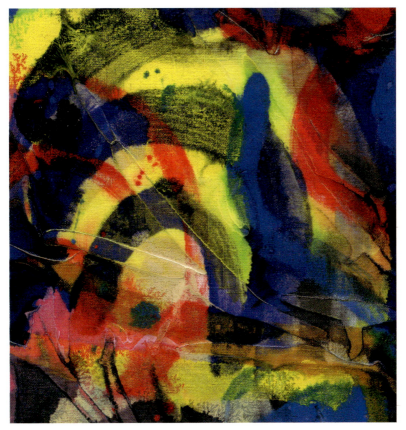

'Abstract'. This is one of a series of artworks made by people with dementia at Fountainsway Hospital in Salisbury.

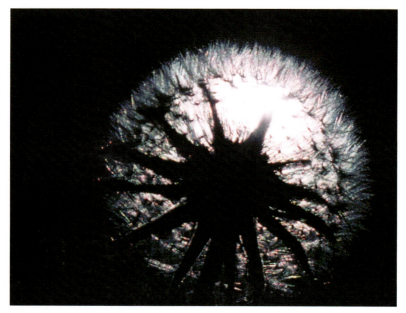

'A Dandelion' by James McKillop. This image is taken from James' book 'Opening Shutters, Opening Minds.' James took up photography following his diagnosis of dementia. Of the image he says, 'To many, dandelions are weeds but if you stay in a place bereft of flowers it would be regarded as a lovely golden bloom.'

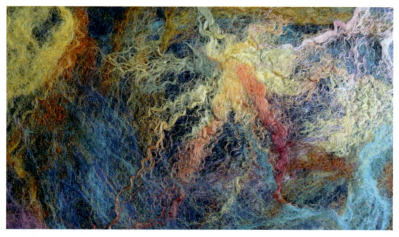

Felt offers an excellent medium for group as well as individual arts activities.

Many of these images featured in the Creativity in Dementia Care Calendars published by Hawker.

PART 3
Making Things Happen

18.
Getting Real

So far in this book we have examined the case for creativity and the arts in relation to people with dementia, and provided examples of many areas in which achievements have already been recorded, and in which opportunities await for those convinced and confident enough to begin to make their own mark in this rapidly developing field of activity. We are now ready to lead you through the practicalities of setting up and sustaining your own projects. But before we do so we need to acknowledge some of the challenges you may be faced with on the journey. We are aware that we have been presenting a very positive view of our subject, and it is only fair that we take account of some of the drawbacks you will encounter and problems you will need to solve to ensure successful outcomes to your endeavours on behalf of, and in partnership with, people with the condition.

Although we must endeavour at all times to see the person not the dementia, we must also take into account the many ways in which dementia can affect our activities. Through proper understanding of these variables we can make subtle adjustments to how we design, offer and facilitate an arts programme in order to create a positive experience and maximise participation.

For example, it is important not to assume that simply making a range of art materials available for a person will be sufficient to ensure that activity takes place. The steps required to begin to engage with a plan can be difficult for some people. Similarly, a person having started may become 'stuck', seemingly unable to pick up an object or move from one stage of a process to another, or they may become trapped in a cycle, repeating the same action over and over again. In these instances it might become necessary to offer a verbal prompt, to help the person to physically take the next step. This might involve placing a paintbrush in their hand, making a mark on a page or guiding a particular action. Gentle music can also offer a natural rhythm and facilitate movement, as can encouraging the person to mirror your actions.

Language can seem to be a barrier. A person may struggle verbally to articulate their thoughts, perhaps forgetting simple words, or substituting one word for another, or talking in a way that you cannot understand. You will be called upon to interpret their communication by other means – by tone of voice, or facial expression, or body language. A person may remain silent, but this does not necessarily mean that thoughts and feelings are not occurring; only that the person may not be able to put them into words, or may be choosing not to do so. We are fortunate that so much, particularly in the visual arts, provides an alternative language to speech.

Then again dementia impacts on short-term memory. This can manifest itself in a number of ways. For instance, a person may struggle to retain simple instructions, to recall who you are, or even to remember taking part in a previous session. Providing written or pictorial instructions, dividing information into bite-sized pieces, and not using over-complicated language can all help. Above all, however, it is important to offer reassurance, recognising how frightening it must feel for a person to be faced with this situation.

Some people may experience disorientation and anxiety. A calm voice on your part, and an unruffled manner can work wonders. If someone cannot settle and begins to leave, and gentle persuasion has not worked, then they should be allowed to go: they are exercising choice. Never forget that there is always a reason for someone's behaviour, even though it may not be obvious to you.

Sometimes it is possible to accompany a person when they are on the move – John has made poems with or sung with individuals in that situation. There are days when someone who on previous occasions has settled to an activity may refuse to participate; a change of mood may even occur an hour or two later and a mutually satisfying interaction or activity can occur. Again, a piece of advice from a person with the condition can be really helpful. Christine Bryden (2005) from Australia offers the following:

> *My stress tolerance is very low and even a minor disruption can cause a catastrophic reaction... I need calm, no surprises, no sudden changes. Anxiety is an undercurrent in our disease. I feel I have to do something but I can't remember what... With the stress of facing many activities at once I become very focused on trying with all the brain I have left to concentrate. Telling me to rest won't help me but helping me to complete a task will.* (Bryden 2005, p.111)

Then there is the vital matter of relationships. There are two aspects to this: the relationship of the person with the facilitator, and the relationship of the person with others (in the family, in the unit, in the group). To take the former, a lot can depend upon the degree of rapport between the two participants in the process whether progress can be made in furthering an activity. Where a clash of personalities occurs then it may not even be possible to get started. It has been our experience that many individuals with dementia develop an acuity which enables them to 'see through' another person and to perceive their underlying motivation. If there is an element of insincerity, or even if there is a lack of confidence in pursuing an objective on the part of the facilitator, this can profoundly affect the outcome. The obverse of this is that when true identification is achieved great things may be possible. In the group situation the facilitator needs to develop skills of amelioration of conflicts as they occur. A mix of abilities can work so long as members are comfortable with each other. New friendships between participants can occur and bear fruit outside as well as within the circle. These are matters we will return to in the following chapters.

How dementia affects the person clearly presents us with a number of challenges. However, even greater is the challenge presented by the wider social/cultural environment and the way the person and their art are perceived. The difficulty is that whatever the individual produces, their work may well be scrutinised through the lens of dementia/the disease. We are dismayed to come across the terms 'Alzheimer's artist', 'Alzheimer's art' and 'Alzheimer's poetry', as if these were discrete categories to be judged by adopting a special critical frame. Claire has worked for some years as a clinician, and in all this time she has never heard the work created by people with musculoskeletal problems referred to as 'arthritics' art' or the work of people with depression as 'depressives' art', so why should we label and evaluate the art works of people with dementia in this way?

Another issue we have encountered is the denial that individuals with dementia can create artworks of exceptionally high quality. As a result, such works are frequently 'explained away' as freaks or the result of a combination of medical factors. As an example of this, Claire recently had a conversation with an eminent gerontologist. She was admiring a set of photographs that a person with dementia had taken as part of a broader project looking at change. When Claire told her about the aims and objects that the works fulfilled the gerontologist dismissed them by saying, 'Oh, he must have such and such a type of dementia and that really doesn't count!'

Sadly this is not the only instance of this type of attitude being encountered.

This raises all sorts of questions when we look at research to support the use of the arts in relation to people with dementia. Again we are faced with a series of dilemmas and methodological questions including: what set of criteria do we measure the outcomes of the work against? Do we focus on wellbeing, on the role of the arts in affirming self-identity and building self-esteem, or do we measure changes in cognition, or in recall? What facet of the art-making process do we particularly address, and how do we record and quantify the changes we observe when dementia may make it difficult for the person to remember or to verbally articulate these experiences? We shall attempt to tackle some of these issues now and revisit these again later in our chapter on evaluation.

19.

Starting Out

In any creative endeavour of this nature the first question you need to ask yourself is 'what is the purpose of this project?' If your response is 'to improve the quality of life of people with dementia' then the next question to ask is 'in what way?' This is important since your answer will effectively underpin the approach taken and shape the direction and substance of the project. Suppose for instance you see the main function of the arts as to provide a source of entertainment. If this is the case it would seem completely reasonable for a project to focus on offering individuals access to a range of performances where they assume a largely passive role as members of an audience. If on the other hand you see the arts and creativity as a vehicle for social inclusion your entire focus and the shape of the project would radically shift. Here individuals would play a very active role and the arts would assume a different function, probably with a community orientation, giving voice.

By inviting you to name or articulate the purpose of the project our intention is not to restrict or limit creativity in any way. The best projects evolve and are shaped by the experiences of those who participate in them. Creativity cannot be contained and as relationships develop and confidence grows in using the arts media new opportunities present themselves and the purpose of the project may move in new and exciting ways. However, stepping back for a moment and thinking about the broader picture, will avoid some of the difficulties we have observed where one facilitator sees the function of the project as creating the work of art and the role of people with dementia as observers of this, whereas others emphasise the expressive qualities of the materials and see the most important aspect as the involvement of individuals in the process of creating.

Time invested in thinking and planning at this point is time invested well; not least, because you may well be asked to present a rationale justifying why your project should take place. We hope to have offered a comprehensive overview of what the arts can offer and painted a picture through worked examples of some of the opportunities they can provide. If you are still unclear as to the range of possibilities you would be well advised to read something of the broader literature and evidence base that supports this work. A good place to start would be a report entitled 'Arts in health: A review of the medical literature' written by Dr Rosalia Lelchuk Staricoff which offers a systematic overview of research looking at the relationship between the arts, humanities and healthcare. The review contains almost 400 references from the medical literature relating to the effects of the arts on health and wellbeing and in the words of the report, *'offers strong evidence of the influence of the arts and humanities in achieving effective approaches to patient management and to the education and training of health practitioners'* (Staricoff 2004, pp.9–10). This document is well worth a read. Whilst the report is medically orientated and does not focus specifically on people with dementia it contains a number of highlights including:

- The value of literature, creative writing and poetry in enabling individuals to *'regain control over their own inner world, increasing their mental wellbeing'* (op.cit p.26) whilst also enabling staff to understand the cultural, social, ethnic and economic factors impacting on how individuals act.

- The potential of theatre, drama and visual arts as vehicles for self-expression and a means through which to promote insight and enable individuals to understand their own world.

- Evidence to support music, singing and dancing as ways of enabling people to recall events from their lives, to express themselves and to increase activity levels leading to improved physical wellbeing.

Some reference is made to the arts in the context of people with dementia including ways that art interventions provide support for both the person with dementia and the mental health professional, and create new approaches to aid the understanding of the condition (Killick 2000; Argyle 2003). Consideration is also given as to how the introduction of the arts into healthcare helps people with dementia to find *'new ways of self-expression and acts as a vehicle for establishing communication with others' (Killick and Allan 1999a; Killick and Allan 1999b; Allan and Killick 2000; Allan 2001)* (Staricoff 2004, p.25).

The importance of music as an aid to support individuals with memory problems comes through strongly. Two studies cited in the report explored the relationship between music and memory. It was found that where individuals were asked to recall particular life events this recall was significantly better in the presence of music rather then silence or noise. On the basis of this work the authors conclude that *'Auditory stimulation by music enhances arousal and attention, helping people with memory problems to remember life events' (Foster and Valentine 2001; Larkin 2001).* (op.cit p.30)

Reference is also made to the use of drama therapy as a way of promoting communication (Snow 2003) and as an outlet for self-expression reflection as a means of aiding understanding (Knocker 2002).

The work concludes by emphasising the value of the arts in increasing self-esteem and supporting the development of positive attitudes and relationships (Smith 1998) and suggests that the *'Creative arts are uniquely suited to the task of preserving and maximising the sense of self in people...mainly because they are non-verbal modalities which encourage self-expression, reminiscence and socialisation' (Johnson et al. 1992)* (Staricoff 2004, p.26).

Whatever the focus, the starting point for this work can be small spontaneous acts of creativity woven into the fabric of everyday routines. You could, for example, take any of the arts media and activities we have described in our book and share these with the individuals you work alongside. Offering a person a pen and piece of paper, sitting with a person listening to what they say, recording this in some way would be an excellent starting point. This interaction might take place over a short period of time and does not necessarily require a specially designated space. It is simply dependent on your willingness to step out and try something new, to approach the person with an attitude of openness and expectation and meet them where they are. To do this you will need to trust the creative process.

In some settings these short bursts of creativity have been sufficient to ignite something much greater and the work has taken on a life of its own, gathering its own momentum. However, these instances, in our experience, are few and very much dependent on the energy and investment of a handful of committed individuals who have carried this forward. To embed creativity within the culture of the environment and realise a broader vision it will be necessary to invest time and energy in planning and creating space where people living with dementia can access opportunities to engage in the arts. What follows are suggestions of ways to plan and implement more systematic projects.

Igniting the creative spark

Start with the bigger picture. Blue sky thinking is required here and at this point don't let the practicalities bog you down. People with dementia are the experts and a key resource in the process. Where individuals struggle to articulate ideas verbally, find alternative ways to listen to their experiences. For instance, artwork, objects, photographs and descriptions of projects in journals and books can provide tangible talking points and offer useful ways to elicit views and ideas when a person finds the spoken word difficult. Family members and colleagues can also offer valuable perspectives and may bring a range of ideas and indicate possible directions of travel.

It might, for example, be that the aim of the work can be met by offering individuals the opportunity to discover and engage in a particular art form such as poetry or dance. The project might accomplish what is required by creating something more structured such as embedding creative sessions within daily routines or could even look outside the immediate environment to build links with the wider community where people with dementia are able to share their skills and draw on wider resources. Or it could be something else. The possibilities are literally endless.

Don't worry too much about the detail at this point. For instance you might feel that creating opportunities to engage in a particular art form will be a focus for the work. It isn't necessary to completely identify what the art form is at this precise moment. That can be saved for later when you know the scope of the materials and resources that are available to support you.

Once you have captured the broader vision, find a way of representing and describing this. Again, you don't have to be too precise. Invite people to name the project by giving it a title so that it is owned by everyone and turned into something concrete. This allows others not directly involved in the process to understand and grasp what it is about. The advantage of beginning with the bigger picture is that it enables you to create a direction of travel, offering a focus and building in some parameters. It is the equivalent of setting out on a journey and identifying the destination or at least having an idea of the country you are travelling to. For one thing it will make the planning process much clearer and for another it will enable you to decide when you have arrived there. It will also give you an idea of the steps you need to take to realise the vision.

The next stage then is to look at the resources you can access as these will also shape the nature of the work. The point about resources is that it might well be possible to introduce a small, spontaneous arts-based project into an environment with little broader support but for this to be sustainable and avoid burnout it is necessary to draw on the skills, time and energy of others.

Use this process to make the project visible. Talk about the work, engage with others and get people on board so that it begins to gather momentum. This is an excellent way to discover some of the hidden facets of people with dementia you are working alongside, to offer individuals a role and draw on their talents which can be considerable. Claire has known actors, musicians, film-makers, prize-winning artists, dancers and published writers all living anonymously in hospitals or care homes. These individuals have animatedly described their interests and generously shared their talents. This has not been limited to people directly involved in the arts – teachers, guide leaders, scenery painters in amateur dramatics societies have all contributed valuable skills to projects.

Family members and staff have also described treasured hobbies or interests that have fed into work. One nurse for instance shared that she had an Open University degree in English Literature and volunteered her time to go on regular outings to the local theatre with residents as part of a drama project. Another carer held a City and Guilds qualification in floristry and offered flower arranging classes for people with dementia living in the home.

Don't limit your search to resources in the immediate environment where you work. Identify resources outside your organisation that you can tap into. Begin with those in the local community: arts groups, local arts colleges for instance, schools, universities, drama societies, churches and faith communities, museums and galleries. Working with such organisations can build a strong sense of community connectedness and ensure that the place where you work is very much part of the environment and valued as such rather than remaining separate.

There are many opportunities here. For instance Claire runs a very successful project where students studying on health courses at the university work on arts-based projects in the local care homes. There are practical considerations, such as ensuring that everyone is CRB checked. However, residents and students value the opportunity to learn from each other and the activity co-ordinators within the care homes appreciate the additional resource and input the students provide.

Anne Davis Basting and John have written an excellent practical guide to developing an arts programme drawing on the skills of artists. They describe a number of models. The approach we've outlined to date would fit the 'facility driven model'. Other approaches include:

- **Artists for hire:** This is where 'an artist is (or artists are) employed to provide the activity for a fixed period and when the time is up the activity ceases.' (Basting and Killick 2003, p.10). The process can be managed by organisations acting as brokers between care environments and artists can be sourced through less formal networks between artists and staff. In the UK, Sandwell Third Age Arts Project is run by the Local Authority where the social services department refers individuals to art-based activity. These are co-ordinated by an administrator who matches the person to the artist. Up to 15 one-hour sessions are then provided in the person's own home.

- **Artist/facility partnership:** Again artists are involved and paid for a designated period of time. However, rather than working independently the artists work alongside staff members, sharing their skills so that the work has a life beyond the immediate duration of the project. This approach has met with success in Scotland. John describes how in one place *'so great was the enthusiasm engendered in the participants that staff (who had also taken part) were able to continue both activities using the knowledge they had gained as permanent elements of the activity programme'* (Basting and Killick 2003, p.12).

Clearly when involving artists there are cost implications and it might be necessary for a number of settings to pool resources, to fundraise or to apply for grants.

There are also a number of national organisations who can provide ideas and support. Magic Me for instance is an organisation focusing on the development of intergenerational creative arts projects. Storytelling, creative writing, photography, weaving, drama, dance, puppetry, carnival, painting and poetry all offer meeting places where young and older people can learn from each other in mutually supportive relationships. The surprising thing you will probably find is that the moment you begin to look for resources others will present themselves, taking you in new and exciting directions you possibly never imagined.

20.

Drilling Down to the Detail

Once you have established the foundations of the project the next step is to work out the practical details. For instance, where and when will sessions take place, for how long? Who will facilitate these? Will the focus be on individual or group? Who and how will you invite people along?

Much depends on the setting, the nature of the creative media, your individual approach and the overall aim of the interaction. For instance, a painting activity undertaken on a one-to-one basis in a person's own home will require a very different set of resources to a group drama session facilitated in a hospital or community setting. The focus, however, whatever the setting and whether group or individual interaction, will always be on the person. It will be necessary to understand where they are at, how they might be feeling, which media might best meet their needs and how you might facilitate this in such a way that they will gain the absolute maximum from the experience.

As part of this process you will need to decide whether you will concentrate on group or individual interaction or whether you will look at a combined approach.

The arts lend themselves well to both individual and group sessions. Groups feed the creative process, taking ideas in new directions and offering participants a sense of togetherness where everyone is speaking a similar language using the materials.

Frequently unpredictable, always sociable, group sessions are perfect for drama, music, some textiles and visual art activities. Individual interactions on the other hand are often more intimate, allowing you to come directly alongside someone and to work very intensively, offering a greater sense of control over the process. Working in this way can help to build confidence where the person is lacking in self-esteem or is physically too frail to engage in a group. One does not preclude the other and where resources are available we would suggest that there is much merit in combining both approaches.

Consideration will then need to be given to where sessions will be held. If a group is planned the space will need to accommodate both the number of participants and the type of activity. The ideal environment will:

- be well lit

- include somewhere for people to sit

- have the option of surfaces to work on particularly if painting or writing

- be sufficiently spacious for everyone to sit with their art work in front of them to avoid feeling overwhelmed and crowded

- have an ambient temperature – a room that is too cold can feel unpleasant and unwelcoming and a room that is too warm will make people fall asleep

- be free from distractions as too much noise can be disabling.

Some facilitators suggest that if arts sessions are occurring in communal settings such as in hospitals or care homes they should be held in a separate room away from shared areas (lounges, dining rooms). This has the advantage of minimising excessive background noise which can be distracting for people with dementia for whom concentration may be difficult. A separate room offers much needed privacy and when this is a designated 'art or creative space' it allows participants to make the association between that space and the activities that take place there. It also prevents participants from leaving en masse in response to external cues. Claire recalls many an occasion where groups have instantaneously dispersed at the mere sound of the lunch trolley arriving on the ward.

However, there can be drawbacks associated with this. For instance it can prevent people with dementia from feeling that they can walk away from the group, have a stretch and return later. It can also be very isolating, excluding other staff and family members preventing them from taking part in the session. Also the reality is that such spaces are an absolute luxury and virtually non-existent in many of the environments we work in. Groups often take place in shared living rooms or at tables in corners of dining rooms. The multifunctional nature of these spaces can be confusing, particularly if someone arrives at a dining room table expecting to eat lunch and is instead confronted by a palette of arts materials. You will need to develop your own creative solutions to such challenges. For instance it might be that during the summer months you access outside areas or find ways of providing visual markers (distinct table coverings) to differentiate group sessions from the usual function of a particular area.

Time and timing are also important considerations. Creativity isn't a switch that can be turned on and off or designated to inflexible blocks of time. Timetables may be used to promote creative work, alerting people to sessions offering a routine and providing a structure, but the ideal is to weave creativity throughout the day so it spills over into (the ordinary) everyday routines. The problem with fixed timetables is that they can become formulaic and not respond to the specific needs of individuals in the moment which is so important for people with dementia who very much live in the 'now'.

Claire recounts an occasion when she was working on an assessment ward for people with dementia and arrived an hour before the timetabled session. She spent time with a few people who were alert, enthusiastic, well-motivated and ready to take part. Staff were concerned that the routine of the ward wasn't interrupted and so Claire headed back to the OT department as requested (*we just like to know where we are with things*). On her return at the allotted time she was met with a completely different picture – the room was silent and people who just an hour before were awake and alert were fast asleep or dozing.

Moving away from a fixed timetable also helps to avoid the 'art in the hour myth' and the assumption that meaningful activities can only occur in substantial chunks of time when the truth is that the duration of group sessions and individual interactions should be completely flexible. Selly Jenny suggests that this is because *Alzheimer's patients have differing attention spans. Some can work only a few minutes at a time*' (Jenny and Oropeza 1993, p.23).

It also reflects the intensity of the creative process and is something we regularly observe in many other sessions we facilitate for artists, staff and students who don't have dementia. Therefore whilst you may plan that your session will run for 45–50 minutes, don't be surprised if it finishes much sooner or runs on much later. It is far better to spend 20 minutes with a person engaging in a quality interaction and stop at the point when they are ready to move on rather than insisting a person stays for a full hour when they are struggling to concentrate. Similarly there is nothing worse than abruptly ending a session when someone is experiencing flow just because the allotted time slot is at an end. If it needs to extend a little, let it be so and build this into your planning. The key is to enjoy the moment and listen to the person so that they tell you when it is time to finish rather than letting the clock dictate the pace of your interaction. Moving away from the art in an hour myth also frees staff to find pockets of time – 10 to 15 minute intervals where short creative bursts with people can occur; spontaneous moments such as singing with someone or sharing photographs, postcards or pictures.

This brings us to resources. We won't say too much about resources here as we have embedded our ideas in earlier descriptions of the arts media. Just to reiterate, good quality materials are a must for any creative session. The materials are a key part of the interaction promoting or inhibiting self-expression, directly impacting on the quality of the end product in terms of what someone can achieve and communicating messages about values attached both to the activity and the individual. This final point is expressed eloquently in the following narrative shared by Sarah Zoutewelle-Morris:

> I remember when my grandmother, a highly cultured Parisian who also composed music and played the piano was in a nursing home. We were at a birthday party with silly hats, treats and music: all this was more suited to a group of five-year-olds rather than the varied adult population present. Grandmère hadn't been communicating much, but at one moment her eyes met mine and exchanged a look with me that said it all, i.e. what a total insult to her intelligence and dignity this activity was. (Zoutewelle-Morris 2011, p.43

In order to avoid such experiences it is necessary to spend time with the person finding out who they are, discovering their interests, past hobbies, roles they have enjoyed. The most successful sessions build the creative activity around the person taking care to understand what might be considered important within the interaction. This is not only in terms of the art form chosen, but also in relation to how the activity is graded to meet the person's needs.

It is often assumed that the most significant factor impacting on this process is dementia. It is true that you will need to take into account how the condition affects a person's concentration, ability to retain instructions or to initiate movement. However, this is only part of the story since physical health, arthritis, poor eyesight, loss of hearing as a result of age can also be disabling. Personality also plays a significant role and can be a key determinant of the direction of travel.

Take for a moment an example: for a time Claire used to paint with a person in a care home called Florrie. Florrie was in her 90s and had dementia which massively affected her verbal communication skills. If Claire visited Florrie in the care home and spent time with her she would withdraw into herself and completely 'clam up', paralysed at some level by self-consciousness.

However, give Florrie a paint brush, a sheet of paper and she was transformed. Claire and Florrie could sit together whilst the paint and conversation flowed. Whilst her speech was still incredibly difficult to follow at times she would find other ways – the title of her painting, the colours she used, the content of the picture. The images were not aesthetically beautiful in a traditional sense, but for Florrie that was not the main concern, it was about the time she spent with Claire, having an outlet for self-expression where she didn't feel self-conscious.

Claire also painted with Erol. Erol was a teacher and after receiving a diagnosis of dementia became incredibly depressed. He still lived at home, but his wife was concerned because he had completely withdrawn into himself and had outbursts of sheer frustration. When Claire painted with Erol the quality of the finished image did count, it was massively important to build his fragile self-esteem. Claire's role within this was to listen and spend time and to find ways to help him achieve the end result he wanted.

To an onlooker Claire would appear to share the same creative activity but the aim, the direction of travel was different. The arts represent a vehicle for self-expression, a shared relationship, a means to build self-esteem, experience feelings of productivity but the emphasis changes depending on the person. For Florrie we are focusing almost completely on the process and the journey, and for Erol whilst the journey is important it is the destination, the end piece that counts.

Each time you work with someone there will be a slightly different focus and your skill as the facilitator is to understand what this is and find a way of building this into the creative activity you offer. Each person will engage on a different level and you may want to think about the materials as:

- a sensory experience

- a story, evoking powerful memories and reminiscences

- a blank canvas for the imagination

- a place for discovery and self-discovery

- an expression of identity and individuality

- building blocks, order, sequencing offering control and choice

- a mechanism to create something beautiful and accomplished, to build and re-build self-esteem

- tools for communication

- a shared space where relationships can flourish

- play.

In some instances the most important element is that the person undertakes the activity independently, in which case it is necessary to ensure that materials are chosen to maximise success. For other individuals it is sufficient to be involved in the process of making or creation and for yet others the act of being present, soaking up the atmosphere, enjoying the company and experience is enough. Every interaction will have a million and one variations of these themes, but each session will have one thing in common which is that at every step of the way the person with dementia is in control. You are merely the co-pilot making those all-important preparations and continual adjustments to make sure the journey is what it needs to be. Most importantly you will learn from the individuals you work alongside the value of relationship and that each person is different. No one moment is ever the same. Clearly then your role within this process is key.

Your role within the process

Selly Jenny states that, *'the overall goal... is to establish a safe haven where the participants will be gently encouraged to use art as another form of creative expression.'* (Jenny and Oropeza 1993, p.12). To enable this to happen, your role as facilitator is to be who the person with dementia needs you to be at that moment in the creative process. Variously you will be supporter, enabler, reflector, engager, encourager, guide, confidante and friend. You will note that we have chosen not to include the word expert here and this is for good reason.

First and foremost, expert denotes power rather that partnership which runs counter-clockwise to the ethos of this book and to any approach of working with people with dementia. Second, it raises the question, expert at what? Being expert at dementia as a condition may help you to understand the challenges a person may face during an interaction. However, being an expert about dementia is absolutely not the same as being an expert about the person and could never replace the importance of coming alongside the individual to find out who they are, to learn about their rich life history, unique personality, likes, dislikes, interests, hopes and dreams.

Similarly being an expert in using creative media would certainly help you to understand the expressive qualities of the materials, to 'tune in' to the language of the arts, the opportunities and challenges they present. Indeed we would argue that:

> *Actors (and artists) have a particular talent for communicating with people with dementia … [that] stems from a quality of attention, concentration, perhaps ability to be still 'in the moment', filtering out all other distractions and claims on attention.* (Benson 2009, p.23)

By the same token there is always the danger that being an 'expert' in using a particular creative medium can distract so the focus shifts to the product, the quality of the finished work rather than resting on the person and their journey.

In both instances, the problem of being 'an expert' is that it can make you closed up, less sensitive to what is happening. The most important element you can bring to any interaction is yourself; your humanity and all this encompasses – personality, life experience, interests and an openness which means that every time you engage in a creative act you are effectively engaging in a process of discovery and self-discovery where anything is possible. Indeed the creative process is about shared relationship, mutual discovery, meaningful making.

Sarah Zoutewelle-Morris expresses this in the following way:

> *I don't see the person with dementia as an imperfect version of someone without dementia. She is a unique individual with a huge potential to surprise and teach me … I am invited to use my creativity to find ways to communicate, validate and support that person where she is as she is. During these encounters I learn to receive as well as give, to be as well as do, and witness as well as intervene.* (Zoutewelle-Morris 2011, pp12–13)

Creativity flourishes in a climate of mutual respect, trust and freedom of self-expression. This requires you to be open, attentive and very much live in the moment. You need to enter into the person's world and meet them where they are rather than expecting them to step into yours. Trust is important here. So is an ability to lose self-consciousness and to go with the flow. We therefore end this chapter with a narrative taken from Claire's book *Meaningful Making* (2003, p.27–28) which captures something of this process.

Sitting on the ward with a blank sheet of paper

It is Monday afternoon and the ward is a hive of activity. Everything seems loud and chaotic, not the usual lull after lunch. A home visit has been cancelled, so I have taken the opportunity to come onto the ward to offer an impromptu arts session. I sit in the dining area with a large blank sheet of paper. Around the paper there is a small selection of pencils, oil pastels, brushes, and small pots of paint.

I speak with Freda and ask if she would like to join me, taking along a visual cue of a small image that she has created in a previous session. However, she seems preoccupied, fingering the sheet of paper, holding it close to her face before screwing up her nose and responding with the words, 'Oh I can't paint love.'

Undeterred I sit down at the table and pick up a pencil, making simple marks on the paper. I am suddenly aware that I am not on my own and Terry is sitting next to me, with a pencil in his hand mirroring the marks that I am making. We do not speak. We don't have to because our marks flow over into each other's space. I mirror his marks back to him. A visual conversation is taking place on the paper where we are making connections, reaffirming each other's existence by the very nature of what we are doing.

Florence looks on. She says, 'He's mine you know,' referring to Terry and I offer her a pencil and ask if she would like to join us. She chooses not to sit but stands and then abandons the pencil in preference for the oil pastel. She sets to work, completely absorbed making huge yellow marks. I offer her another colour and she takes the blue and starts to work again. Terry stops to watch and then we are joined in turn by Enid and by Arthur who ask what we are doing. Florence seems most put out and tells us that she is drawing her garden. I ask her if we can help and she nods her head, sitting down, tired from the effort. As she sits Terry stands and walks away from the table.

Enid struggles to make a mark so I ask her if she would like me to draw with her. She tells me that she would like to see a dog in her garden and we talk a little about home and how it feels to be away from things.

Arthur doesn't need any assistance. For a moment he is engaged deep in conversation with Florence speaking in a language that I cannot understand. Yet each is completely absorbed by what the other is saying. Florence has taken control and Arthur is making marks now in accordance with her directions.

Suddenly I am aware that Terry has returned and with him he has brought Freda who looks on.

Visitors have started to arrive and the dining room suddenly feels chaotic. Enid's family have arrived with her granddaughter. Enid hasn't noticed and my signal for them to join us has been politely turned away. They just seemed pleased to see her absorbed in the activity. From the corner of my eye I see her granddaughter whispering to her mother and instinctively I ask if she would also like to join us. For a few wonderful moments granddaughter and grandmother draw together and there is a meeting of worlds.

The sound of the tea trolley echoes down the corridor. The magic is broken and the group disperses. I sit back to admire the work and marvel again at the simplicity and the power of the materials. Personally the blank sheet of paper represents a meeting place on the ward where individuals can express their creativity, their hopes, fears and wishes. It is a space where the only agenda is that of the person with dementia and where it is not necessary to do but sufficient simply to be.

21.

Giving Creativity a Shape

Creativity takes many forms and moves in any number of directions. As the previous narrative has shown the nature of this, its tempo is directed by the person so that at times it can resemble a dance with the person with dementia taking the lead. As a consequence, creativity is never formulaic or contained. However, as a rule, most creative sessions will comprise some kind of shape. Whilst we are never quite sure about where an activity will lead, most of the individual and group interactions we are involved in loosely consist of an invitation, a beginning, middle and an end. Here we begin to unpick these elements in more detail.

Interactions begin with invitation. When a person's self-confidence is low and they are fearful of making mistakes, the act of engaging in any form of creative activity can feel risky and frightening. Careful consideration needs to be given to how to ask a person to join you since the invitation to 'come to paint' or 'write' or 'sing' can feel threatening and the response, 'I can't do that' or 'not today' can belie a deeper lack of confidence rather than a genuine wish not to take part. Visual prompts or a sharing of materials can be helpful here, a gentle introduction, a reminder of who you are and a warm greeting can give the person confidence to take the first step. As Selly Jenny writes, the person needs 'a place to regain a sense of belonging, a gentle environment within which to combat this feeling of loss and insecurity' (Jenny and Oropeza 2003, p.5).

Beginnings

Beginnings then need to be about welcome, reassurance and establishing the meeting as a safe place to be. This is the point from which everything else flows. It requires you to be completely present in the moment, to pause for a second and to look. What do you see? What do you feel? What do you notice about a person's non-verbal communication? Is the person or group relaxed, uncomfortable, nervous, annoyed, angry? How do you feel? Imagine just for a second that nothing exists beyond the events that are unfolding before you. This will enable you to be responsive.

Claire describes how she spends time planning sessions, preparing the room beforehand so that she can focus on the person rather than fussing over resources. However, over time she has learned that the first few moments of the interaction determine its direction, its flow. If she enters a room and people are anxious or agitated her response is soothing, reassuring. If the group is tired, unsettled or distracted then the tempo is upbeat, exaggerating the intention to engage, to capture and hold attention. She begins with a clear plan, a shape of the session in mind, but with the knowledge that following those first few moments this may quickly be abandoned, changed and redeveloped to meet the needs of the person or the group in the here and now. Here she describes her approach to the beginning of her group sessions.

I like to indicate that our time will be distinct and special. To this end I mark the beginning in some way. This might be something as simple as turning off a television, closing a door or introducing a ritual or routine. I might play music to greet people, wear a distinct scent or a particular item of clothing to act as a reminder of who I am. Once we are together I turn the music off and welcome each person by name, creating an anchor point and offering an opportunity to gain a sense of how the group is feeling. We then talk about the activity, exploring objects or pictures as tangible prompts, eliciting memories, sharing experiences and building relationship. If I am working with a person on a one-to-one basis we might spend a little time exploring the environment together and the materials that are in it.

Middles

What follows then is time and space to engage with the materials. Choice is important here but too much choice can be paralysing and offering one or two options is preferable. If instructions are required, these are simple, uncluttered, shared at appropriate moments and based on the understanding that too much information offered at once can be overwhelming and confusing. Visual prompts, photographs depicting stages of the process and lists of instructions are all helpful. If the needs of the person or group are significant we will work alongside individuals to begin the process of 'creating together' before stepping back and letting the person engage in the act of making. Sometimes we might demonstrate elements of the process. Claire for instance usually participates in some form of art making as a way of modelling a technique so that others can feel confident they have 'permission' to do the same. Time and timing are of the essence and the greatest skill is an ability to read the situation since to dive in and support someone at too early a point can undermine confidence and leaving them to struggle on their own can risk the person giving up and walking away.

Endings

Sessions are always relaxed and the person or group sets the tone. As individuals complete what they are doing or begin to tire we pause and prepare for an ending to the interaction. Endings are all about celebration. There is usually a moment when we stop and reflect, admiring what has been created, sharing something about the process. It is at this point we thank everyone for coming. Again a closing ritual can be helpful. For instance drama therapist Paul Batson (1998, p.20) describes how at the end of his drama sessions he invites participants to link hands, look around the group and say 'thank-you' to one another as a means of reinforcing the sense of a shared experience. We have also found it helpful to include an element of re-orientation since the person is often moving from a place where play, improvisation and imagination are encouraged to an environment where emphasis is placed on reality, accuracy and memory. For this reason it can be useful to talk about what is happening in general, focusing on everyday things such as 'what's for tea' before returning with the person to the space beyond the session.

Beyond the session

Making sure that arts materials are properly cleaned and stored will help them last longer. Within group situations, the act of clearing away can form an activity in itself. It has a magnetic quality that draws people in. If the group has taken place in a communal area people sitting on the periphery will often appear with offers of help. Dementia can rob people of important life roles – wife, husband, mother, father, housewife, provider. The simple act of clearing away can restore a sense of self. One person said to Claire, *'Oh I have enjoyed that, it makes me feel just like a person.'*

The final piece

Here is a short extract taken from Claire's reflective journal of the experience of painting with a person with dementia:

The abstract image is tiny. Swirls of magenta and vermillion intermingled on the water colour paper. Rich, delicate. It represents a meeting between Margaret and myself. Each line has been considered. Initially the marks were faltering as she tried out the materials, gained a sense of the paint, exercised choice, selected the colours, mastered the brush. The final layers are richer, more definite, a tribute to her growing confidence. In the very early sessions she would watch as I sat during my break with my scraps of watercolour paper, making marks... In time I have discovered her wicked sense of humour, a real sense of fun which she expresses in so many ways – a huge splodge in the middle of an otherwise ordered piece. Her rebellion. Sometimes all I gain is a sense of her frustration as she scribbles over the paper with frantic marks. Fast pace, fast rhythm, intense, absorbed. On other occasions she is weary, tired, disinterested, making tiny feint marks which I mirror back to her on the paper... after I have gone the painting will be there as a concrete record for all to see of a journey that we have travelled together, the joys and frustrations that we have shared in trying to express ourselves through the language of paint. (Craig and Killick 2004, pp.193–194)

There is a sense that work produced and what it represents lives beyond the interaction. The question of what happens to a person's work is an important one. Valuing the work created by a person with dementia is about valuing the person who has created it. This might be something as simple as framing a painting, recording a song, typing up a poem, photographing an image and presenting it back to the person who is the rightful owner of the work. The work always belongs to the person, it is theirs to do with as they will and if there is any suggestion of the artwork being shared more broadly you must first seek the person's consent to do so.

22.

Measuring Success

Evaluation is an ongoing process that enables you to compare what you thought would happen with what is actually going on. This is helpful because it allows you to recognise what is working well and include more of this and identify what is working less well and include less of this. When undertaken appropriately, evaluation provides a space for people with dementia to reflect on their experiences, giving voice so that individuals can play an active role shaping the project and effectively become co-designers or partners in the process. It can also be a source of motivation for you and the individuals you are working alongside and create tangible evidence of what this approach has to offer. This can be useful if you need to justify staff time and resources to support the ongoing work.

However, whilst the reasons for evaluation are extremely sound, the process is not without challenge. For one, *'Responses to art are of such a personal nature'* (Basting and Killick 2003, p.26). The main difficulty then lies in part in deciding what to measure and how to measure this. For instance will you measure an aspect of the creative process or the quality of interaction? Might the emphasis be on the degree to which creativity supports cognition or increases wellbeing? What about the way creativity compensates for some of the more insidious effects of dementia on the person for instance by reducing social isolation, improving self-esteem, promoting communication? Or perhaps you will look at something completely different, for instance the quality of relationships, attitudes of staff or carers towards the person.

In some instances the focus may be dictated in part by the setting in which you work and its broader philosophy and will tap into elements of a much more fundamental debate relating to the purpose of the arts which on the one hand sees creative expression as a form of treatment and on the other as a basic human right and a key component of wellbeing. Either way you will need to identify your stance and recognise the complexity of capturing and recording this.

During the planning process you might want to consider evaluation in relation to what you hope the project will achieve in the long term as well as looking at more immediate gains. Long-term objectives focus on the bigger picture considering how the creative approach we describe leads to tangible gains for the individuals you work alongside over time. You may choose to concentrate solely on people with dementia (e.g. increased confidence, development of defined roles, increased opportunity for communication and the formation of relationships, opportunity to engage in pleasurable activities, develop hobbies) or encompass broader changes within the setting where you work (for instance in the culture of the environment, increased interactions between staff and people with dementia, shifts in attitude). Short-term objectives on the other hand describe the more immediate effect of taking part in arts-based interactions and can again relate to both people with dementia and the experiences of others sharing in the process.

It can be useful to develop these at the beginning of your project as they can set the tone of what you hope to achieve and reinforce the direction of travel. Again the process should be seen as essentially creative offering rich opportunities for collaboration and expression. We can both think of examples where this has been exceptionally successful. For instance one person Claire worked alongside chose to paint a picture to capture what they hoped to gain from taking part in the art group they were part of.

This was then used as a concrete representation of the standard against which each session was then measured.

Clearly measurement is an important consideration and it will be necessary to identify a series of indicators that will enable you to demonstrate the degree to which the project met individual expectations/you achieved what you set out to do. Much depends on your focus. The types of measures you might use to look at wellbeing, for instance will be very different from those used to demonstrate improved concentration. We have included signposts at the end of the book to articles describing a range of tools. Here are a few examples of our approach to evaluation:

Sharing experiences

Make evaluation an integral part of the activity as opposed to an add-on. This might be something as simple as providing space for participants to comment on their experience, identify things they have enjoyed or not enjoyed or compare feelings at the beginning of the interaction with feelings at the end. Do not underestimate the ability of individuals to articulate their experiences and to describe what the arts have offered. Increasingly we are seeing a number of rich accounts describing the benefits of creativity written by people with dementia (Friedell 2001; McKillop 2003; Bryden 2005 for instance).

Where verbal communication is difficult word cards, symbols or images to indicate responses can be helpful. Sets of cards containing descriptive words (fun, boring, difficult, childish, interesting) or 'feeling words' (this activity made me feel: relaxed, tired, upset, happy, loved, calm) offer a structure or scaffold which individuals can use to organise their thoughts as well as providing 'permission' to talk about things they have found difficult or would like to change. Kate Allan in her excellent work exploring the experiences of people with dementia utilised a range of still images, inviting people to choose an image that best reflected how they were feeling (Allan 2001).

Comments and responses can then be noted or recorded in some way. Better still, invite the person to use the arts materials as the medium for evaluation. The piece might take the form of a poem, a performance, a photograph, a song, a painting or another representation to express or capture something of how it has felt to be engaged in the session. This can be accompanied by a verbal description although frequently the work is sufficient to convey the quality of the interaction and can offer a visual or verbal narrative to map out the high points and low points of the creative journey. The finished pieces speak volumes and avoid the dissonance that can sometimes occur when the experience of participating in an act of making/creating is measured by a linear questionnaire.

For individuals at a more advanced point in their dementia, you may need to rely on more observational methods. Dementia Care Mapping is one example of a tool that offers a way of measuring the wellbeing and illbeing of individuals in group settings although training is required to use this. Less formal techniques may include noting people's responses during an interaction or the use of video, sound recording or even still photography to capture specific moments. Arlene Astell has used video to great effect when evaluating the creative use of technology (Astell *et al.* 2010). For any method using observation, and particularly for those involving photography or video, it is always necessary to gain permission from participants prior to a session.

Finally do not underestimate the value of your own reflections on the process. Again these may take the form of written accounts, drawings or photographs capturing something of the experience. Claire uses a technique of 'play-back' where she tries to imagine the session from the perspective of a participant in order to gain an alternative view of events and then writes about this. Journalling is another useful way of recording experiences providing a good reference point when looking back and reviewing sessions. Where groups are facilitated with carers or staff, such reflections may take the form of verbal discussion based around shared observations of the process.

Sometimes after a planned number of sessions have been offered it can be useful to pause, gain an overview of the experience and to look at the opportunities and challenges the programme has offered. Questionnaires and interviews are two methods that can be used to access this information. Questionnaires help you to build a broad picture whilst interviews offer rich, detailed accounts enabling you to 'drill down' to the specifics. Anne Davis Basting and John explore this issue of evaluation in their book about the arts. They emphasise that people with dementia may have difficulties in recalling their experiences and suggest that the following methods can be useful in prompting recall:

Showing extracts from videos.

Playing sound-recordings of sessions.

Showing photographs of sessions.

Showing props/tools/artifacts used or made in the sessions.

Showing evaluation cards (Basting and Killick 2003, p.26).

The best methods of evaluation are those which are flexible and responsive to the situation. Less beneficial are those that are so narrow that they focus on a set of immovable, inflexible, pre-defined criteria that blinker everyone to what is happening before them. Here is an example from Claire's work to illustrate what can occur when a narrow approach is adopted:

I was working in a setting using an arts-based approach. As part of this I spent time with each person discovering their strengths and interests, seeking to understand their needs in order to build up a picture in relation to what the arts might offer, establishing individual and general goals against which I could evaluate the work. With these elements in mind I was able to ensure that sessions were designed in such a way as to open up opportunities for all those involved. The project went well, moving in new, exciting but unexpected directions. The evaluative elements were flexible enough to accommodate these changes since they looked at the quality of engagement within sessions as well as exploring changes in relation to the overall wellbeing of participants through observation. As a consequence the overall evaluation was an honest reflection of what had occurred within the group, its strengths and limitations. However the hospital had recently developed a set of outcome measures against which every intervention was judged. These measures focused on changes in relation to physical, cognitive and psychological function. Not only was the process of 'administering' these to group members extremely disempowering, but the tools were insensitive to small changes and as a consequence showed little or no change in participants' cognitive functioning. Based on this information, in spite of all the evidence demonstrating increased interaction, communication, engagement and expression of humour, the project was seen of little value...

This experience throws up all kinds of questions, not least relating to the validity of the measures used. Whilst the setting fully embraced Tom Kitwood's (1993) model of person-centred care recognising that we are far more than the sum of our cognition, it chose to use a measure that simply failed to look beyond this. This is a salutary tale about the importance of choosing an appropriate evaluation tool.

Reporting/sharing findings

Finally, once you have captured the experience, understood the overall impact of the project and weighed up its strengths and limitations, it is important to give consideration as to how this will then be presented and shared. Whilst there is a growing recognition that creativity has much to offer people with dementia, there is a sense that we need to share our learning, to highlight ways of gaining the most from the arts to develop even more ways of working with the media. In this way the approach will evolve and grow.

If you work within an organisation there may be certain rules and regulations in terms of with whom and how you can share the findings. You may be expected to present your evaluation in a particular format; for instance in a report or as a presentation. However, if you do not operate within these constraints this process of reporting can be an important part of the overall project, generating feedback, creating interest and acting as a springboard for the development of subsequent projects As Anne Davis Basting writes:

> *Sharing the work that emerges in art programs can be a powerful way to reach out to families, staff and the community at large.* (Basting and Killick 2003, p.29)

Celebrating the work, sharing the opportunities and challenges presented gives voice to and celebrates something of the people who have been part of this. Central to this is the involvement of people with dementia. For example, at the end of a very successful residency, John invited people who had been part of this work to participate in a reading of their poetry. The experience was powerful and exceptionally moving as people with dementia were able to share their work and to speak of the life-transforming effect of the experience on their lives. The audience which included family members, external organisations and the funders of the work could be left in no doubt of the value of the project. Indeed, video, photography, poetry readings and art exhibitions are all vehicles through which projects can be shared. The principles of permission and ownership described in previous chapters clearly stand. However, the strength of these media is that they offer immediacy, a level of engagement, a tangible record of the experience, a platform for future work and a means to enable the work to live on.

23.

Making Space for Your Own Creativity

Making space for your own creativity is absolutely central to the success of any arts project. First and foremost, you are valued. If the arts and creativity can offer people with dementia the opportunity for meaningful expression, an outlet for emotion, a way to think about and reflect on experience and increase self-esteem, doesn't it also make sense that the arts can offer all these things to you? This might be in relation to your confidence or the coping mechanisms you employ to manage some of the pressures of balancing work and home. Working alongside people with dementia is an immense, enriching experience but it demands that you make yourself completely available and this requires you to draw on all your emotional as well as physical reserves. Working so intensively without the means to express and work through some of these feelings can lead to exhaustion, depression and ultimately burnout. We both know all too well how it feels to have given your all to the point that you are running on empty. Creativity can be restorative because it offers space to get in touch with, process and work through some of these feelings. Baines describes this in the following way:

> *Those trained in the psychoanalytical tradition... would say that creative acts connect us to our unconscious and allow us to draw on resources and strengths, which a person may not believe that she or*

he has at her or his disposal... what is known is that being creative, whatever happens to us, is good for us. It assists in keeping our brains functioning well. (Baines 2007, p.9)

There is a growing body of evidence to support this. For instance in a study undertaken by Repar when care staff working with people with dementia explored their creativity through massage, yoga, music and writing, participants experienced significant reductions in levels of stress (Repar and Patton 2007). The literature identifies further possibilities. For instance, Anne Davis Basting writes,

When we express ourselves creatively, we learn something about who we are. By adding something new to the world we also add something new to – and grow – ourselves. Finally through creative expression we share ourselves and connect with others. (Basting 2003, p.8)

The arts offer an opportunity to gain new insights and experience personal growth. One of the ways they do this is by helping us to revisit what we thought we already knew and experience the world at a more intuitive, sensory and emotional level. First and foremost this can promote empathy offering the means to *'use the senses to grasp feeling, stretch the imagination to see a new perspective and ... enhance understanding'* (Peloquin 1996, p.655).

When we are no longer bound by logic we are more open to new possibilities and what might be. This means that we are more receptive to the individuals we work alongside and more able to work in the moment, since everything in some ways is a potential opportunity to enable the person to become. Perhaps this is one of the reasons why through creative expressions *we are so able to connect with others* because our minds are not closed to the possibility of doing this. This closely mirrors the process described by Tom Kitwood (1993):

As we discover the person who has dementia we also discover something of ourselves. For what we ultimately have to offer is not technical expertise but ordinary faculties raised to a higher level: our power to feel, to give, to stand in the shoes of another through the use of our imagination. (Kitwood 1993, p.17)

Whatever the mechanism, the arts offer a form of communication that is not dependent on words. Given that conversation is a two-way process, it is important that you engage with the materials in order to understand the qualities of media, to grasp their expressive potential and effectively learn something of this language and all that it has to offer. This will help you to understand a person's response, to experience how it feels to be confronted by the material and to build your confidence and understanding of ways of working with this. In understanding the nuances of the media you will be able to gain the most from your creative interactions and be more in tune with how a person might be communicating. Ultimately this could offer a far greater depth to the creative interactions and the quality of the relationships you develop will be richer because of this.

Finally there is a practical argument for building confidence in using the materials. Experiencing a sense of familiarity and mastery with regard to the media can help you to feel more confident when sharing these with others. This can be helpful as people with dementia are often tuned into emotion and will pick up very quickly if you are feeling stressed or confused. Your confidence will be soothing and will inspire others to feel confident.

We hope we have presented a good argument here as to why you need to make space for creativity, now we turn to how.

Creativity is not just a set of activities you engage in or something you do. It is as much a way of being: playfulness, an attitude and way of looking at the world. As you have read this book and experimented with different media you may already have found different media that you have 'connected' with or found yourself wondering 'what if...' Have there been times recently or in the past where you have found yourself exploring or playing with the materials? We have a theory that we don't 'find' creative media, they 'find us' and once you begin this creative journey it doesn't stop. The starting point of this process is to give yourself permission to do this. You need to make a commitment to engage in some form of creative engagement for at least 20 minutes a day. Twenty minutes is probably less than it takes you to drink a cup of tea, but it offers a starting point if the thought of making time just feels too daunting. It can help if you allocate a space for this to happen or even a time that you schedule in. Otherwise it can easily disappear. Claire keeps a small sketch pad where she keeps a visual diary and a reflective log, a record of an ongoing journey.

If this leaves you cold and you still feel at a loss in terms of where to start, we have found the following exercises very useful to get the creative juices flowing:

- Visit a local gallery.

- Enter 'creativity' or 'the arts' into a search engine on the Internet and see where this takes you.

- Wear something a bit different.

- Set yourself a creative challenge.

- Try something new.

- Buy a doodle book and give yourself permission to play.

- Try different ways of signing your name: develop a new signature.

- Go on a walk and as you do identify an object you connect with.

- Buy Betty Edward's book, *Drawing on the Right Side of the Brain* and follow some of those activities.

- Go to a conference on the arts, creativity and dementia.

- Buy a copy of the *Journal of Dementia Care* or *Signpost*.

- Go to the dementia positive website http://www.dementiapositive.co.uk/

- Have a look in your local paper for classes involving art, drama, dance or other creative media and go along to one, just for a try.

- Read any of the books on Claire or John's bedside tables (full details in the list of References).

Books on Claire and John's bedside tables

Betty Edwards: Drawing on the Right Side of the Brain
Antoine de Saint-Exupéry: The Little Prince
Christine Bryden: Dancing with Dementia
James McKillop: Opening Shutters, Opening Minds
Susan Sontag: On Photography
John Killick: You are Words

Brian Keenan: I'll Tell Me Ma: A Childhood Memoir
Sara Maitland: A Book of Silence
Holly J. Hughes (ed.): Beyond Forgetting: Poetry About Alzheimer's Disease
Manjusvara: The Poet's Way
G. Allen Power: Dementia Beyond Drugs: Changing the Culture of Care
Douwe Draaisma: Why Life Speeds Up As You Get Older

Whatever the starting point, the good news is that creativity feeds creativity. Embarking on this journey may initially feel a little strange or alien but as you trust the process and your imagination flourishes you will discover untold opportunities and possibilities. We promise, you will not be disappointed.

PART 4
Living It Out

To date, we have presented a range of creative media and looked at the practical steps required to introduce some of these ideas into the setting where you work. In this final part of the book we offer a series of short narratives to illustrate how our ideas can be translated into practice across a range of contexts considering some of the opportunities and challenges this presents.

24.

All Together

The Arts as Identity

Claire Craig

Sessions can be concentrated around a particular medium, but this needn't always be the case. This is an example of where art, writing, drama and drawing were used within a project focusing on life-story work in a long-stay environment for people with dementia.

Cedars was a 30-bedded unit for people with dementia. A recent inspection had flagged up the need for a more focused approach to activities and I was invited to help in the planning of a project. Having spoken to residents, carers and staff it was clear that there wasn't in any sense the feeling of 'community'. The high turnover of care assistants made continuity difficult. New staff, many who did not have English as a first language, were struggling to understand who people were and this had increased the anxiety levels of family members who felt that the needs of their loved ones were being neglected.

Although there was in theory a timetable of activities, because there was neither a budget nor a group of people who were committed to this component, they often fell by the wayside. If staffing was problematic such sessions were frequently the first thing to go. However, my impression from the outset was that in spite of very difficult circumstances, staff were completely committed to the residents and that they were very keen to see activities taking place on the unit.

The greatest need it seemed was in offering individuals a space to learn about each other. When I initially suggested life-story work to the manager she dismissed this outright because of concerns in relation to resources and the difficulties of organising regular sessions. She was also unsure as to how her overworked staff might feel in relation to another pressure that would be placed on them. However, following assurances that this would not be the case she fully gave her support and so the project began.

The work began with a single invitation to people living on the unit, their families and staff. It read:

Telling your story

We all have a story to tell. Over the next four weeks we would like to invite you to tell yours. Come along to our workshops and individual sessions and discover how to do this. The workshops are open to everyone and will be advertised on the notice board. Watch this space.

We started small with a story-wall. The unit had a long corridor and we created a time-line of dates and events in history. The question, 'Where were you then?' invited people to write, draw or pin pictures to the board. Because the dates went right up to the present grandchildren could also participate. The activity quickly gathered momentum and very soon the story-wall began to be populated so that it resembled a very large collage, with pictures and sheets of paper containing reminiscences spilling over. Visitors would admire the board, taking time to read its contents and showing a genuine interest in the information it contained. Some staff contributed to this process and it was interesting to read these accounts. There were also a couple of occasions when I noticed staff were using the wall as a focus, pausing with residents as they walked people to and from the bathrooms, leading to impromptu reminiscence sessions.

A family member brought in a map of the local area and people began to mark on streets where they lived, the local schools attended. It wasn't always factual, sometimes individuals living (and working) on the unit constructed intricate stories reflecting more the life they would have liked rather than the reality. These stories were incredibly telling. Such was the success of this that we extended this to a world map. Again, we simply pinned this to a board and people indicated places they had travelled by using different coloured stickers. Some staff described this as an epiphany when they recognised the extraordinary rich lives people had led. We also built a number of creative activities around this. For instance, 'wish you were here' was an activity using photographs and images of places. People with dementia, families and care staff were invited to choose an image and imagine they were sending this as a postcard to a friend or family member. Very simply they shared what they would have written. The poems and prose that followed were extraordinary – poignant and happy, filled with memories and dreams... Originally intended as a group activity, it spilled over – daughters shared this with mothers, grandparents with grandchildren, husbands with wives. 'Finding my way back home' was the title of one particularly memorable piece.

Two further elements concluded the first stage of this approach. The first was an invitation to choose five objects that were important to the person. The objects couldn't be living and they needed to be able to fit into a shoe box. Improvisation was the name of the day. So, for instance if a person valued a particular piece of furniture, a dolls' house model would suffice. This was very revealing. Tiny pairs of bootees, a set of keys, a small prayer book, letters, poems, lots of photographs all found their ways into the boxes. We encouraged everyone to take part and there was energy as some people (not everyone) chose to share what their boxes contained and all the resonances that naturally emerged. Family members said that they had particularly appreciated the opportunity and that it had been a very powerful shared activity. The lesson was that this needed to be treated with sensitivity. In the words of a member of care staff who recently took part in a similar exercise, *'I felt as though the essence of who I was had been captured in a series of objects.'*

The second element was a writing project based around the theme 'These I have loved'. We based this on an idea shared by Deborah Philips, Liz Linington and Debra Penman in their book *Writing Well* (Philips *et al.* 1999). They suggest a simple writing structure based on the senses where individuals are invited to think about a favourite view, scent, texture, sound and taste and can represent this in any way they choose. Some individuals for instance chose images, for others it formed the basis of a piece of creative writing or an art activity and this work was undertaken within workshops on the unit. Again, everyone was invited to attend.

At this point we reviewed the work to date, seeking out feedback from people with dementia, staff and family members. The most encouraging element was that individuals didn't just speak about having fun and the process of creating they spoke of learning about each other. There was a real sense of people coming together, sharing and feeling part of something bigger. Not everyone chose to take part. *'Work is work and what I do in my own time is my own business'* was a response from some staff and these views were respected.

Not everything succeeded either. I had an idea to include more around drama and creative play, inviting people to select an item from a suitcase of clothes something they felt best represented their personality. This quickly disintegrated into a jumble sale as people chose things they would like to have. It was an enjoyable process but not quite what I had in mind. I also tried to encourage family members to write short accounts, memories of the person seen through their eyes. Only one person did this and she spoke of it being a most moving experience, but I simply ran out of time to take this further. The time I had been allocated for the project had come to an end although it did feel a natural place to leave things.

I was part of planning the next step and I respected the decision that the focus would now be on helping individuals to construct their life-stories, making handmade books of images and text. I felt this would work well and there was certainly enough momentum, but I did have reservations in terms of how these might take shape and whether they would be left unread, locked away in bedside cabinets. You see above all, experience taught me that the value of the approach was in finding points of connection, identifying those details that encouraged the development of relationship. This approach worked so well within the unit because it brought people together. The great advantage of using a range of media was that everyone could be involved and the connections could take place on multiple levels, offering a depth and richness to the process that I had previously not encountered.

25.

Beyond Grass

Claire Craig

It was an inauspicious start to say the least. More concrete than landscape. But that was the beauty. It was a 30-foot square blank canvas and ours. Well that it how we saw it at least; a starting point with the potential to offer much to individuals who attended the unit. Access was important. People were physically frail or reliant on using a wheelchair to move around and consequently would have struggled with steps. Luckily the area could be accessed down a gentle slope with a grab-rail to the right making it relatively easy to come and go. Once this was established, seating was therefore our first priority. Another occupational therapy department at the hospital offered help and people attending a heavy workshop as part of their rehabilitation began crafting beautiful wooden benches and bird tables, believing that if birds regarded this as a garden area then it was indeed a garden.

This was where creativity took hold. Everyone had an idea about what a garden was and needed to include. We had the vegetable/flower debate and the water feature/no water feature discussion and there was a flurry of activity as people brought in nature magazines, pictures of childhood gardens and reminisced about their own plots. There were some fabulous stories: unexploded bombs in back gardens, marrows the size of beach balls, the battle of the moles and other tales. It was also an opportunity to learn about how people from different countries regarded these spaces. Take for instance Maria who was from Spain where the outdoors was Siesta, and Sangria and Aleksander from Poland for whom the outdoor space was farming and survival.

I did try to introduce some sessions where I invited people to draw out their ideas, but the unit offered predominantly individual sessions with people and this was difficult to co-ordinate. Consequently it was easier to invite people to bring along objects they would like to include in the space to make it theirs. This proved to be very successful and the fun was trying to find a purpose for the most obscure pieces. Someone brought a series of old clay pipes, for instance, which we turned into a raised bed, packed with flowers and herbs. A leaky hose became a water feature and a bag of old forks and spoons a wind-chime. Imagination knew no bounds and neither did people's generosity, donating cuttings and seeds enough to fill a hundred plots.

And so this space evolved. Everyone played a part in its making and because of this it was used in different and wonderful ways. For some it was about the opportunity to plant and grow and to nurture. For others it was about having the space to walk or sit in the fresh air, to relax, watch the birds or play. For each person the place took on new meaning, a blank canvas for the imagination. There were moments. For instance the time when Frank planted the seedlings only to be followed by Alice who dug these up as part of her 'weeding,' but these moments were just part of the outdoor experience.

The placement was short and I moved on. Had I stayed I think we would have thought about the evenings, ways of involving the community, perhaps exploring the potential for intergenerational activities or ways of bringing music into the space.

The experience made me reflect on the creative potential of the outdoors and challenged my thinking in terms of what I regarded as a garden. It wasn't conventionally beautiful, a real hotch-potch, but I believe that this was part of its appeal. So often when you think about gardens in the context of creativity and people with dementia you think of perfect designs, beautifully executed which can carry the message of 'you can look but don't touch'. There can be the assumption that for a space to work it is necessary to employ landscape designers, build expensive features. We hope that this narrative has gone some way to challenging this assumption. Our space was a blank canvas for the imagination, chameleonic in nature and most importantly the act of bringing this into being was undertaken in partnership with the people for whom it was intended making the process itself a creative act.

26.

Two Residencies
The Dream and the Nightmare
John Killick

This is an account of two pieces of work, contrasting in every way: one extended in time, the other brief; one covering a wide geographical area, the other in one part of an institution; one involving a large number of people, the other very few. In other ways these two were poles apart, as I shall explain. What they had in common was that they were both writing projects, with similar objectives: to give a good experience to the participants; to encourage others to become involved in the work; to have worthwhile end-products; and to counter stigma through demonstrating what people with dementia can achieve when the right stimulus is provided.

The first project was countywide. The money had come from the National Health Service, but was organised by the local library service. A big plus-point in the first project was the amount of planning that preceded the start of the project proper: lists of possible partner organisations, individuals with an interest, and venues where the work might be carried out. Attractive publicity material was drawn up and distributed. Follow-up phone-calls were made. Library staff were mobilised to transport me from place to place to make the maximum use of the time available.

The statistics alone are impressive: over 25 contact days I worked in six day centres, nine nursing homes and one hospital ward. I saw 77 people with dementia in one-to-one sessions, and 127 in groups, and 294 staff in training sessions, whilst 232 members of the public came to talks and readings. I gave six readings in libraries, made two broadcasts, and a book and a calendar were produced; some were distributed and a large number sold. The total cost was £15,000.

I can only sum up this residency by saying that it was like a dream. Everything worked, and allowed me to concentrate on building relationships and making poems. I have many memories of creative encounters with individuals and with groups, and I left behind tangible records of what was achieved in the book and calendar, both of which are still circulating in the community. Here are two comments from participants:

> *This is heaven, because for a lot of people it helps them. You do it as a one-to-one and that's right. I feel I'm very lucky because I've got something like poetry.*

> *You've made me try and use my brain in a way no-one else here has, and I thank you.*

The second project was held in an assessment ward in a local hospital. The money came from the Friends of the Hospital.

The statistics from this second project read rather differently.

Over 10 days I worked with five residents, ran two training sessions for staff but four attended, only one of whom worked on the unit. The only outcome was a display board in a corridor on which poems were mounted. The cost was £3000.

No prior planning appeared to have gone into this residency. Few relatives had been contacted for permission for me to work with those being assessed. On the day before I arrived, the manager was transferred to another post, and a temporary manager was put in, who was ignorant of the project and unsympathetic to what I was trying to do. There was also a new overall manager of the mental health units, and he started on the same day as me. Two half-days of training had been arranged and, as I have already indicated, only one person from the unit came: she was already keen on my appointment and remained an enthusiastic supporter throughout. The second session of training had to be cancelled for lack of support.

One of the ideas of the manager who was transferred was that my presence would in some way encourage best practice on the ward. The situation was that as staff did not know why I was there they could not support me, so for most of the time I was left to my own devices. I introduced myself to two relatives when they visited and shared with them the work that had been produced. I worked there two days a week for five weeks, and there was a considerable change from week to week in the clients available, probably 25 to 30 persons in total. However, I only had permission to work with five of these, so many people missed out on the opportunity to create poems. The general atmosphere on the ward was unpropitious for any kind of creative activity, and I found myself having to force myself to go to the unit in a morning. I was not surprised when one staff member said to me: *'Is this the worst place you have ever worked? And if you say "No" I won't believe you.'*

The experience of being involved in these two projects in quick succession highlighted for me the crucial nature of pre-planning and proper support during the event. The lack of these ingredients creates the conditions for a dream or a nightmare for the facilitator, is the difference between bringing benefits to the community or an institution, and can either constitute a wise investment or a waste of money.

27.

Putting on the Ritz

Claire Craig

Putting on the Ritz was the rather splendid title chosen by a group of care staff to describe a drama project based around creativity and mealtimes. The idea came about during discussion of some of the barriers they faced in making time for arts-based projects in the setting where they worked. The feeling was that time was of the essence with little opportunity for formal groups or sessions. If it was impossible to create extra time we moved to thinking about ways of using existing time, focusing particularly on the fixed everyday routines of bathing, dressing and dining. When we looked at these we realised that each offered an extraordinary number of opportunities. For instance dressing was all about choice, self-expression and identity. Bathing opened up opportunities in relation to relaxation, play, sensory stimulation. However ultimately the group settled on food and mealtimes simply because when we started to look at this the scope and potential seemed endless.

And so the project was born. The group wanted to bring a touch of class to the dining experience which they felt was rushed and mechanistic. The decision was made to turn the clock back to the days where scones and jam were part of the everyday and reinstate the institution of afternoon tea. Some staff were sceptical, others felt they lacked confidence and would struggle to do this. We therefore hit upon the idea of turning this into a drama project where each person could take on a 'role' and play a part 'in character'. Time was spent considering the environment where this would take place. It was felt that it needed to be distinct. Someone suggested that if this was a drama there needed to be some kind of set with props. This sparked lots of ideas as another person remembered that there were nice tablecloths and 'posh crockery' at the back of one of the cupboards. Someone else offered to dig out a cake stand and doilies and another person said they would bring in music and a CD player. The final question then was what to wear. This generated the most debate but ultimately it was decided that in the spirit of the event black skirts and white aprons were the order of the day!

I wasn't privy to the actual event, but by all accounts it was a massive success. The staff animatedly recounted each minute detail: who was there, who responded to what, how one of the residents suddenly took on the 'role' of staff and started serving tea and another person began to dance to the music. The overall feedback was how enjoyable the experience had been for everyone and whilst it was felt that the black skirts and white aprons would only appear on special occasions, the music, ambience, and the idea of stepping into a role had made this into something very special, a living out of the creative process that could take place on every day of the week.

28.
Ian and 'Me-ness'

John Killick

Some years ago the BBC approached me to make a radio programme about how I made poems with people with dementia.

This is how I came to meet Ian. At the time he was 59 years old and living with his wife in a small town just outside Glasgow. I went there seven times over a period of three months with my recording equipment. Out of this material I made eight poems, only one of which was used in the programme. I see this as a distinctive body of work, which gives us unique insights into dementia and one individual's struggle to retain command of his intellectual processes.

When we started working together Ian told me that he hated poetry: the way it had been studied at school had put him off. I told him to leave the poetry side of things to me: he was just to say what was on his mind at any time.

Ian, though highly sensitive, was a straight-talking, feisty individual. He would have no time for small-talk but go to the point at once. I would arrive at his flat, set up the tape-recorder and get down to business. He would stride around the room, talking rapidly and fluently, and getting increasingly excited – he would often kick the microphone over in his enthusiasm. I would respond to occasional questions and remarks but tried not to interrupt the flow. There was considerable banter between us, and I believe that was a significant factor in the success of the collaboration.

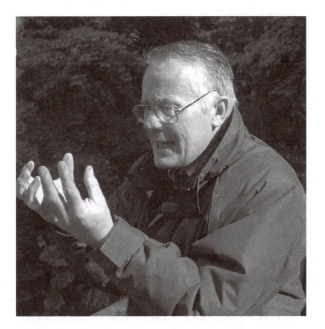

Ian McQueen

Occasionally Ian would suddenly lose the thread of what he was trying to say. Once he trailed off in mid-sentence and said: *'Look, the little creature, it's running along the skirting-board and disappearing with my thought!'*

I would take the tape away, draft any poems I could shape from it and bring them back to Ian at the next session. His usual response was amazement, succeeded by pleasure. Sometimes he expressed disbelief that he had said these things, and I would have to replay the tape to prove that the poem had indeed been made out of his words and thoughts. Once he rejected a poem: *'No good. It has only one four-letter word in it'*. That defect was easily rectified: we put some more in.

Here is one of Ian's poems:

The Slitherer

If I were an artist
I would make a big snake-like thing,
slithering about like that,
getting away back down
into the depths, right down
into the bottom, and there
it would be.

And it's got
plenty of time, so it waits
and it waits and it waits.
Till there comes a time
when this sonofabitch
creeps up on me and says
'I'll stiffen you pal.'
And then it's away again.

In most of his poems Ian personified Alzheimer's as malign: Big Al. In *Defence* he went back to his childhood. The comparison is with a particular school bully whom he had stood up to. He says that the lesson he learned stands him in good stead in coping with what Big Al throws at him today. The style is forthright, slangy even, and typifies his no-nonsense approach. The poem, as well as the incident described, packs a punch:

Defence

Bobby was bigger than me.
And when I got it, I got
a right good thwack from this bloke.
He just ladled into me,
and I couldn't stotter, I was
lying in the playground. Biff! Out.

Bobby was going to get a doing.
And I administered it.
If you steam into me: Stars.
I cloaked myself in my self

and that was good for me.
I got that from him too.

I had my dose,
and Bobby had his dose.
Big Al's bigger than me too,
but I'm not going
to lie down under his blows.
He's in there. I can still
cloak myself in my self.

When the programme was made, and Ian was satisfied with his part in it, I asked him again what he thought of poetry. He replied:

A poem is something that feels into my psyche. It is where it comes out and where it ends up – essence of essences. What matters to me is the me-ness of it.

29.

Alan

A Quick-Change Artist

John Killick

In Chapter 7 I described The Funshops and how they affected the participants. Here I introduce one person who benefited greatly from the provision.

On the first occasion this group met Alan attended, but his body language suggested he would rather be elsewhere. The session began with coffee and introductions. When it came to his turn Alan described himself with reticence and modesty. He stated:

> *I'm here because of my wife. I don't want to be here. She made me come. She thinks it will be good for me. I have never been to any social event since I was told I have this dementia thing.*

I did my best to make him feel welcome, but he seemed acutely uncomfortable. Despite his protestations, I included him in all the exercises and sketches. In a brief chat over lunch he vouchsafed to me that he was an amateur painter. I asked him if he would bring some photographs of his pictures to our next session. When he left, though, I wasn't at all sure that I would see him again.

On the occasion of the second meeting of the group Alan arrived a quarter-of an-hour before anyone else, and settled down to talk to me. He still protested that he was there under duress, but it was obvious that he was pleased to have a one-to-one. When the others arrived he brought out photographs of his paintings and described how he had done them. This resulted in general expressions of admiration. Alan took part in the exercises more readily than on the previous occasion, but when it came to the sketches he began complaining again. However, we now saw this as more like a comedian spinning a yarn rather than a genuine grievance and began pulling his leg, a practice he seemed to enjoy.

I thought up a special sketch we could do together and put him in charge of the improvisation. He was the artist and I was the client commissioning him to paint my portrait. As my demands grew ever more absurd he kept a straight face and accepted all the conditions imposed. At the end he turned to the rest of the group and, with a twinkle in his eye announced, *'I do not accept this commission.'* Everyone fell about laughing and his timing and control played a significant part in this. Afterwards he said to me, *'You're sending me up,'* but there was no reproof in his voice. When he had gone I reflected that he had spoken more than anyone else in the session as a whole.

At our third meeting Alan was again early, and showed enthusiasm to interact with others as they arrived. He played a full part throughout and laughed a great deal. At the end we had ten minutes to spare and I asked the group what we should do. Alan immediately stood up and addressed the group:

> *I want to say something. When I first came here I didn't want to come. My wife sent me. But I found everyone so friendly and it was easy to join in. This is only my third visit and my attitude has completely changed. And that applies to things outside as well. I had only wanted to shut myself away and not see anybody. Now I am going out shopping and I have joined a club and I don't mind who I talk to. I put it all down to what we do here.*

When everyone had left the development officer who organises the sessions said:

I have never seen such a positive change in any client in such a short time. Alan seems a different person.

It is difficult to know how much of this can be attributed to the social aspect of the occasions, but I am convinced the activities of the Funshops, the improvisations and the humour engendered, played a significant part in Alan's transformation.

30.

Painting with Olivia

Claire Craig

I had known Olivia all my life. As the mother of my best friend Julie she had been privy to most of the trials and tribulations that I had faced as a teenager and throughout all these times had been a rock. She was an intriguing character, as colourful as her name, bringing a taste of the exotic to Yorkshire. For one thing she smoked and drank sherry in the afternoon. She wore bright scarves and liked to paint. She had also been known, on occasion, to consult a medium to find out about her future and whether there was another man somewhere on the horizon as wonderful and romantic as her husband who had sadly died. I liked her a great deal. She added a splash of colour to an otherwise grey landscape which I think you need when you are 14.

Exams came and went and in spite of promising to keep in touch at university, Julie and I went our separate ways. Years later, when I was all grown up and working for an archive service, we bumped into each other in the middle of a supermarket on the edge of town. She invited me for tea but then added apologetically, *'Mum will be there.'* *'Great,'* I responded, *'it will be good to see her.'* My friend hesitated, *'She's not the same. She has dementia.'* The statement didn't particularly register; it was long before my training to be an occupational therapist and I'm not even sure if I knew what dementia was but I do remember saying very simply, *'It will be wonderful to see you both.'*

When I went to visit, Olivia didn't remember my name, but as I sat with her she stroked my hand and fiddled with my ring as in the old days. *'Do you still paint?'* I asked. *'Oh no,'* Julie responded on her behalf, *'that was a long time ago although I have kept some of the paintings in the loft if you'd like to see them.'* This was the starting point of our painting together. I would go once a fortnight with my sketch-pad and a small box of watercolours and we would sit and paint while Julie went out and juggled the millions of other things she needed to do. I'm not a classical artist, so I found Olivia's silences reassuring. I just really enjoyed being with her watching her work, more vibrant and daring as ever with random strokes of purples and vermillion. It was as though the more she physically shrank and retreated into herself the bolder artistically she became. She was all there on the page, mischievous, full of surprises and the exotic. The images were scenes from the past, the cuckoo clock from Jersey, even the funny little one-eyed pug whose name defeats me made some sort of appearance although I suppose that in knowing her, I knew what I was looking for. When she had enough of painting she would just stop. Then we'd sit together and eat chocolates and I would tell her about work and she would sit with her eyes closed listening.

Julie said that when she spoke to her Mum after my visits she didn't remember anything about what we had done together but that her Mum was more confident, more at peace with herself and that she noticed that she had taken more of a pride in what she wore. I don't know if this was true, but it was interesting that when I didn't visit because of holidays Julie said that her Mum would be strangely agitated, looking through the window as though she was expecting someone to come.

Olivia went into a care home and I visited a few times with my sketch-pad and chocolates, but the home was noisy and I found the experience too upsetting especially on one visit where her fabulous long grey locks had been cut and permed. The staff suggested that my presence was too upsetting, and although I sent her a card at Christmas and on birthdays I never went back.

I didn't know anything about dementia then and knew probably even less about painting, but I knew Olivia and have frequently looked back on this time with incredibly fond memories. When you sit and paint with someone you form a spiritual connection that goes beyond words, to the point where you can anticipate exactly how they feel and what they need. It is a wonderful feeling. I began painting with her as a favour to Julie, but in truth I continued because I wanted to do it for me and it was this encounter that renewed my interest in art and painting and ultimately led me on the path to be an occupational therapist.

Whilst writing this I found myself wondering whether if I had met Olivia after my training things would have been any different. Sadly I suspect that they might have because I would have been more mindful of the condition, might possibly have wanted to bring along various aids and adaptations and would probably have been more conscious of interpreting her actions through the lens of dementia.

Why have I shared this narrative? Lots of reasons. I suppose in one sense the textbooks can slightly sanitise the arts, using the term in relation to treatment or making it slightly inaccessible. At one point whilst writing this I found myself trying to think of ways that would have justified that our time together was productive when the truth of the matter is that with anyone who doesn't have a label of dementia it would be enough just for that person to enjoy an interaction and simply be. It is hoped that the narrative also illustrates something of the richness of spending time with a person wherever they are sharing the same creative space.

Conclusion (And a Beginning)

We can't attempt to sum up the subject-matter of this book. Like any map it covers a lot of ground. And we are aware that what we have offered you, our readers, is really only a sketch-map, with the detail to be filled in by yourselves (and ourselves) in further forays into the territory. But we hope we have convinced you that this is a journey well worth taking.

We are conscious of what we have left out. There are artforms and activities which, for reasons of space, have received barely a mention, together with good people working in the field of whom we are aware (and no doubt some of whom we are unaware) who are absent from the text. We have not aimed at total comprehensiveness.

There is one area, however, which deserves special highlighting here because of its importance and its difficulty of accomplishment, and that is creativity in individuals with advanced dementia. We are neither of us keen on dividing dementia into 'stages', but we have in mind those who perhaps could be considered in the palliative care time of their lives. Health may be severely deteriorated and communication through the spoken word of extreme difficulty. It is our conviction that the arts have still much to offer those in this condition. Although we have not labelled them as such, some of the approaches outlined in Part 2 of the book can retain a relevance to such people.

But we also need to develop new ways of engaging them and fresh means of evaluating their responses. Apart from the key communication strategies of maintaining eye-contact, touch, etc we can read to people, show them pictures, give them objects to handle, and sing or play music to them. The effects of allocating time and consideration in these ways can be mutually rewarding, but to date it is a neglected area and there is little to report in the way of research or first person accounts to enable us to establish guidelines for practice. This is a challenge which we fervently hope to see soon being met.

We end with a brief extract from a song which John heard someone singing on a unit; the words and music would appear to have been made up by the singer:

> *O World, I don't know what to do*
> *I want to see my sunset*
> *I want it as it was promised*
> *I'm waiting for the hour*
> *I want to see my sunset good.*

References

Allan, K. (2001) 'Communication and consultation: Exploring ways for staff to involve people with dementia in developing services.' Bristol: The Policy Press. Available as a PDF from www.jrf.org.uk/publications/exploring ways-staff-consult-people-with-dementia-about-giving-services

Allan, K. and Killick, J. (2000) 'Undiminished possibility: The arts in dementia care.' *Journal of Dementia Care 8*, 3, 16–21.

Argyle, E. (2003) 'Art for health: The social perspective.' *Mental Health Nursing 23*, 3, 4–6.

Astell, A. J., Ellis, M. P., Bernardi, L., Alm, N., *et al.* (2010). 'Using a touch screen computer to support relationships between people with dementia and caregivers'. *Interacting with Computers, 22*, 267–275.

Astley, N. (ed.) (2003) *Staying Alive: Real Poems for Unreal Times.* London: Bloodaxe Books.

Baines, P. (2007) *Quality Dementia Care. Nurturing the Heart: Creativity, Art Therapy and Dementia.* Australian Government: Alzheimer's Australia.

Basting, A.D. and Killick, J. (2003) *The Arts and Dementia Care: A Resource Guide.* New York: The National Centre for Creative Aging.

Batson, P. (1998) 'Drama as therapy: Bringing memories to life.' *Journal of Dementia Care 6*, 4, 19–21.

Benham, L. (2008) 'A sensory stairwell.' *Journal of Dementia Care, 5*, 16–17.

Benson, S. (2009) 'Ladder to the moon: Interactive theatre in care settings.' *Journal of Dementia Care 17*, 20–23.

Berger, J. (1992) *Keeping a Rendezvous.* New York: Vintage International.

Bergson. H. (2006) quoted in Gunn, J. A. Bergson and His Philosophy. South Carolina; BiblioBazaar.

Block, H. (1998) *Herblock: A Cartoonist's Life.* Connecticut: Easton Press.

Boal, A. (1979) *Theatre of the Oppressed.* London: Pluto Press.

Boal, A. (1992) *Games for Actors and Non-Actors.* London: Routledge.

Boal, A. (1995) *The Rainbow of Desire: The Boal Method of Theatre and Therapy* London: Routledge.

Brough, B.S. (1998) *Alzheimer's With Love*. Lismore, New South Wales: Southern Cross Press.

Brown, S. Gotell, E, Ekman SL (2001) 'Singing as a therapeutic intervention.' *Journal of Dementia Care 9*, 4, 33–36

Bruce, E. and Schweitzer, P. (2008) 'Working with life history.' In M. Downs and B. Bowers *Excellence in Dementia Care*. Maidenhead. Open University Press.

Bryden, C. (2005) *Dancing with Dementia*. London: Jessica Kingsley Publishers.

Cappeliez, P., O'Rourke, N. and Chaudhury H. (2005) 'Functions of reminiscence and mental health in later life'. *Aging and Mental Health 9*, 4, 295–301.

Carr, I., Jarvis, K. Moniz-Cook, E (2009) 'A host of golden memories.' In E. Moniz-Cook and J. Manthorpe (ed.) *Early Psychosocial Interventions in Dementia*. London: Jessica Kingsley Publishers.

Clarke, A., Hanson, E., Ross, H. (2003) 'Seeing the person behind the patient: Enhancing the care of older people using a biographical approach.' *Journal of Clinical Nursing, 12*, 697–706.

Coaten, R. (2007) 'Exploring reminiscence through dance and movement.' *Journal of Dementia Care 9*, 5, 19–22.

Coker, E. (1998) 'Does your care plan tell my story? Documenting aspects of personhood in long term care'. *Journal of Holistic Nursing. 16*, 435–52.

Cooper M.C. and Barnes, M. (1995) *Gardens in Healthcare Facilities: Uses, Therapeutic Benefits, and Design Recommendations*. Martinez, CA: The Center of Health Design.

Craig, C. (2001) *Celebrating the Person*. Stirling: Dementia Services Development Centre.

Craig, C. (2002) *Creative Environments*. Stirling Dementia Services Development Centre.

Craig, C. (2003) *Meaningful Making: A Practice Guide for Occupational Therapy Staff*. Stirling Dementia Services Development Centre.

Craig C. (2005) *Focusing on the Person: Exploring the Potential of Photography for People with Dementia*. Dementia Services Development Centre, Stirling University.

Craig, C. and Killick, J. (2004) 'Reaching out with the arts: Meeting with the person with dementia.' In A. Innes, C. Archibald, C. Murphy (ed) *Dementia and Social Inclusion*. London: Jessica Kingsley Publishers.

Czikszentmihalyi, M. (1996) *Creativity Flow and the Psychology of Discovery and Invention*. New York: Harper Perennial.

Czikszentmihalyi, M. (2008) *Flow: The Psychology of Optimal Experience.* London: Harper.

Day, K., Carreon, D. and Stump, C. (2000) 'The therapeutic design of environments for people with dementia: A review of the empirical research.' *The Gerontologist 40,* 4, 397–416.

De Saint-Exupery, A. (1974) *The Little Prince.* London: Pan Books.

Department of Health (2007) *Report of the review of arts and health working group.* London. Department of Health.

Draaisma, D. (2006) *Why Life Speeds Up As You Get Older: How Memory Shapes Our Past.* Cambridge: Cambridge University Press.

Edwards, B. (1993) *Drawing on the Right Side of the Brain.* London: Harper Collins.

Edwards, H. and Chapman, H. (2004) 'Contemplating, caring, coping, conversing: A model for promoting wellness in later life'. *Journal of Gerontological Nursing, 30,* 16–21.

Eno-Daynes J (2000) *Pathways – Communication and Dementia* Newsletter. June/

Fay, G. (1995) Available at www.bangor.ac.uk/imscar/dsdc/data/The%20 Creative%arts3, last accessed January 2011.

Foster, N.A. and Valentine, E.R. (2001) 'The effect of auditory stimulation on autobiographical recall in dementia.' *Experimental Ageing Research 27,* 3, 215–228.

Friedell, M. (2001) *Dementia Survival: A new vision.* Available at http://morrisfriedell.com/Vision.htm, accessed 1st July 2011.

Gersie, A. (1991) Storymaking in Bereavement: Dragons Fight in the Meadow. London: Jessica Kingsley Publishers.

Gibson, F. (2004) *The Past in the Present: Using Reminiscence in Health and Social Care.* London: Health Professions Press.

Greenland, P. (2009) 'Dance: Five-minute love affairs.' *Journal of Dementia Care 17,* 1, 30–31.

Haq, S. and Zimring, C. (2003) 'Just down the road a piece: The development of topological knowledge of building layouts.' *Environment and Behavior 35,* 1, 132–60.

Henri, R. (1923) *The Art Spirit.* Philadelphia; J.B. Lippincott.

Hill, H. (2001) *Invitation to the Dance.* University of Stirling: Dementia Services Development Centre.

Hill, H. (2003) 'A space to be myself.' *Signpost 7,* 3.

Houston, A. (2009) 'Making things more real.' *Journal of Dementia Care 17,* 6, 20–21.

Hughes, H. J. (2009) (ed.) *Beyond Forgetting: Poetry and Prose About Alzheimer's Disease.* Kent. Kent State University Press.

Hughes, P.C. and Neer, R.M. (1981) 'Lighting for the elderly: A psychobiological approach to lighting.' *Human Factors 23*, 65–85.

Jarvis, K. (2001) *Collage and Dementia: A Practical Guide for Carers and Care Workers.* London: Alzheimer's Society.

Jenny, S. and Oropeza, M. (1993) *Memories in the Making: A Program of Creative Art Expression for Alzheimer Patients.* CA: Alzheimer's Association of Orange County, California.

Jerrome, D. (1999) 'Circles of the mind.' *Journal of Dementia Care 7*, 3.

Johnson, C., Lahey, P. and Shore, A. (1992) 'An exploration of creative arts therapeutic group work on an Alzheimer's unit.' *Arts in Psychotherapy 19*, 4, 269–77.

Keenan, B. (2010) *I'll Tell Me Ma: A Childhood Memoir.* London: Random House.

Killick, J. (1997) *You are Words.* London: Hawker.

Killick, J. (2000) *Openings.* London: Hawker.

Killick, J. (2000) 'The role of the arts in dementia care.' *Nursing and Residential Care 2*, 12, 572–4.

Killick, J. (2003) 'Funny and sad and friendly: A drama project in Scotland'. *Journal of Dementia Care 11*, 1, 24–26.

Killick, J (2008a) 'It moves you, it hits you inside. Reading Poems at Redholme.' *Journal of Dementia Care 16*, 6, 28–29.

Killick, J. (2008b) 'Museums, the arts, responsive care and supportive design.' *Journal of Dementia Care 16*, 4, 24–26.

Killick, J. (2009) *The Elephant in the Room.* Cambridgshire Libraries.

Killick, J. and Allan, K. (1999a) 'The arts in dementia care: Tapping a rich resource.' *Journal of Dementia Care 7*, 4, 35–8.

Killick, J. and Allan, K. (1999b) 'The arts in dementia care: Touching the human spirit.' *Journal of Dementia Care 7*, 5, 33–7.

Killick, J. and Allan, K. (2001) *Communication and the Care of People with Dementia.* Maidenhead: Open University Press.

Killick J. and Rose S. (2002) *Art for the Person's Sake.* Stirling: Dementia Services Development Centre.

Kitwood, T. (1993) 'Discover the person, not the disease.' *Journal of Dementia Care 1*, 1, 16–17.

Kitwood, T. (1997) *Dementia Reconsidered: The Person Comes First.* Buckingham: Open University Press.

Knocker, S. (2002) 'Play and metaphor in dementia care and drama therapy.' *Journal of Dementia Care 10*, 2, 33–7.

Larkin, M. (2001) 'Music tunes up memory in dementia patients.' *The Lancet* *357*, 9249, 47.

Lee, H. (2006). 'Weaving memories and dreams'. *Aged Care* Australia Magazine, April, 22–23.

Lovell B., Ancoli-Israel S., Gevirtz R. (1995) 'Effect of bright light treatment on agitated behavior in institutionalized elderly subjects'. *Psychiatry Research, 57*, 7–12.

Maitland, S. (2008) *A Book of Silence.* London: Granta.

Manjusvara, (2010) *The Poet's Way.* Cambridge: Windhorse Publications.

Matthews, C. (2003) *Pattern and Mosaic in the Garden.* London: Hamlyn.

McCloskey, J.L. (1990) 'The silent heart sings'. *Generations Winter*, 63–5.

McKeown J., Clarke, A and Repper, J. (2005) 'Life story work in health and social care: Systematic literature review'. *Journal of Advanced Nursing, 55*, 2, 237–47.

McKillop, J. (2003) *Opening Shutters, Opening Minds.* Stirling: Dementia Services Development Centre.

Miles, M. (1994) 'Art in hospitals: Does it work? A survey of evaluation of arts projects in the NHS.' *Journal of the Royal Society of Medicine 87*, 3, 161–3.

Miller, B.L. (2000) 'Functional correlates of musical and visual ability in frontotemporal-lobe dementia.' *British Journal of Psychiatry 176*, 458–63.

Mitchell, R. (2005) *Captured Memories. A Photography Project in a Drop-In Centre.* Stirling; Dementia Services Development Centre.

Montgomery-Smith, C. (2006) 'Musical exercises for the mind.' *Journal of Dementia Care 14*, 3.

Moos, I. and Bjorn, A. (2006) 'Use of the life story in the institutional care of people with dementia: A review of intervention studies.' *Ageing and Society 26*, 3, 431–54.

Mullan, M. (2005) 'Finding harmony together through musical expression.' *Journal of Dementia Care 13*, 2, 22–24.

Murphy, C. (1994) 'It started with a seashell: Lifestory work and people with dementia'. Stirling: Dementia Services Development Centre.

Murphy, C. (1995) 'This is your life'. *Journal of Dementia Care*, March/April, 9–11

Nakamura, J. and Czikszentmihalyi, M. (2005) 'The Concept of Flow.' In C.R. Snyder and S.J. Lopez. *The Handbook of Positive Psychology.* Oxford: Oxford University Press.

Olds, S. (2009) Quoted from Woman's Hour, BBC Radio 4 27/08.

Passini, R., Rainville, C., Marchand, N. and Joanette, Y. (1995) 'Wayfinding in dementia of the Alzheimer type: Planning abilities.' *Journal of Clinical and Experimental Neuropsychology 17*, 6, 820–32.

Peloquin, S.M. (1996) 'Art an occupation with promise for developing empathy.' *American Journal of Occupational Therapy 50*, 8, 655–61.

Perry, J. (1997) 'The rich texture of memories.' *Journal of Dementia Care 5*, 4, 16–17.

Pietrukowicz, M.E. and Johnson M.M.S. (1991) 'Using life histories to individualise nursing home staff attitudes towards residents'. *The Gerontologist, 31*, 105–6.

Philips, D., Linington, L. and Penman, D. (1999) *Writing Well. Creative Writing and Mental Health.* London: Jessica Kingsley Publishers.

Podhoretz, N. (2005) quoted in Cohen, G.D. *The Mature Mind: The Positive Power of the Aging Brain.* New York. Basic.

Powell, H. and O'Keeffe, A. (2010) 'Weaving the threads together: Music therapy in care homes.' *Journal of Dementia Care 18*, 4, 24–28.

Power, G.A. (2010) *Dementia Beyond Drugs: Changing the Culture of Care.* London: Health Professions Press

Rentz, C.A. (1995) 'Reminiscence: A Supportive Intervention for the Person With Alzheimer's Disease.' *Journal of Psychosocial Nursing, 33*, 15–20.

Repar, P.A and Patton, D. (2007) 'Stress reduction for nurses through arts in medicine at the university of New Mexico hospitals.' *Holistic Nursing Practice 21*, 4, 182–186.

Rose, L. and Schlingensiepen, S. (2010) 'Meeting in the Dark; a musical journey of discovery.' *Journal of Dementia Care 9*, 2, 20–24.

Rose, L. *et al.* (2008) 'Music for life: A model for reflective practice.' *Journal of Dementia Care 16*, 3, 20–23.

Rutherford, F. and Burns, J. (2008) *Knitted Lives.* Exhibition Catalogue. Gateshead. Equal Arts.

Sacks, O. (2007) *Musicophilia.* London: Picador.

Shipway, E. (1999) 'Creating a life story book'. *Alzheimer's Disease Society Newsletter*, February 4.

Sloane, P.D., Mitchell, M., Preisser, J.S., Phillips, C., Commander C., and Burker E., (1998) 'Environmental correlates of resident agitation in Alzheimer's Disease Special Care Units.' *Journal of the American Geriatric Society 46*, 862–9.

Smith B.H (1998) 'Literature in our medical schools.' *British Journal of General Practice. 48*, 1337–1340.

Snow, S., Damico, M., Tanguay, D. (2003). 'Therapeutic theatre and wellbeing', *Arts in Psychotherapy, 30*, 2, 73–82.

Sontag, S. (1977) *On Photography*. London: Penguin.

Staricoff, R. (2004) *Arts in Health: A Review of the Medical Literature*. London: The Arts Council.

Teresi J.A, Holmes D and Ory M.G (2000) 'The therapeutic design of environments for people with dementia: Further reflections and recent findings from the National Institute on Aging Collaborative Studies of Dementia Special Care Units'. *The Gerontologist, 40*, 4, 417–21.

Topo, P., Outi Mäki, O., Saarikalle, K., Clarke, N., *et al.* (2004) 'Assessment of a music based multi-media program for people with dementia.' *In Dementia 3*, 331–350.

Ulrich, R.S. (1992). 'How design impacts wellness', *Healthcare Forum Journal, 35*, 5, 20–25.

Ulrich, R. and Zimring, C. (2004) *The Role of the Physical Environment in the Hospital of the 21st Century*. New York: Robert Wood Johnson Foundation.

Winterson, J. (2010) The Guardian Review Section 08/05 p. 3

Zoutewelle-Morris, S. (2011) *Chocolate Rain: 100 Ideas for a Creative Approach to Activities in Dementia Care*. London: Hawker Publications.

Further Reading and Resources for Specific Topics

Seeing a bigger picture

The following books are useful if you want to understand more about dementia, how it impacts on the person and ways of thinking about the condition.

Bryden, C. (2005) *Dancing with Dementia*. London: Jessica Kingsley. [This is a first hand account of how it feels to live with a diagnosis of dementia. If you want to learn more about dementia this would be an excellent place to start].

If your focus is on best practice in working with individuals the following books have much to offer.

Downs, M. and Bowers, B. (eds) (2008) *Excellence in Dementia Care*. Maidenhead: Open University Press.

Kitwood, T. (1997) *Dementia Reconsidered: The Person Comes First*. Buckingham: Open University Press.

Marshall, M. (ed.) (2005) *Perspectives on Rehabilitation and Dementia*. London: Jessica Kingsley Publishers.

Key texts for practice

The following recommendations are excellent reads if you aim to understand key issues impacting on people living with dementia and ways of promoting wellbeing.

Basting, A.D. (2009) *Forget Memory*. Baltimore: John Hopkins University Press.

Killick, J. and Allan, K. (2001) *Communication and the Care of People with Dementia*. Maidenhead: Open University Press. [This is essential reading].

Marshall, M. (ed.) (2003) Food, Glorious Food: Perspectives on Food and Dementia. London: Hawker.

Marshall, M. and Kate Allan, K. (eds) (2006) *Dementia: Walking not Wandering – Fresh Approaches to Understanding and Practice.* London: Hawker. [This is extremely readable and offers fresh approach to understanding and practice in relation to this important area].

Zeizel, J. (2010) I'm Still Here: A Breakthrough Approach to Understanding Someone Living with Alzheimer's. London: Piatkus Books.

If you are interested in reading more about different types of evaluation the following articles may be of interest.

Moniz-Cook, E., Vernooij-Dassen, M., Woods, R., Verhey, F., *et al.* For the Interdem group (2008) 'A European Consensus on outcome measures for psychosocial intervention research in dementia care'. *Aging and Mental Health.* *12*, 1, 14–29.

Staricoff, R.L. (2006) 'Arts in health: The value of evaluation. *The Journal of the Royal Society for the Promotion of Health, 126*, 3, 116–120.

The arts and people with dementia

Schweitzer, P. and Bruce, E. (2008) *Remembering Yesterday, Caring Today.* London: Jessica Kingsley Publishers (this book exemplifies a thoroughgoing and creative approach to using memory in a European-wide context).

Zoutewelle-Morris, S. (2011) Chocolate Rain: 100 Ideas for a Creative Approach to Activities in Dementia Care. London: Hawker.

DVDs

I Remember Better When I Paint is a DVD produced by Artists for Alzheimer's in America. The main body of the film is about group visits to Museums and Galleries, but there are a number of other features included in its 52 minutes. To purchase visit www. artistsforalzheimers/whenipaint.html

Fountains Jolly Inn is produced by STAA (Sandwell Third Age Arts), and traces the development of a project in a care home in which a social area was transformed into a bar through the creative talents of the residents. It can be downloaded from www.staa.org.uk

There is a Bridge is a DVD produced by the Memory Bridge Foundation in Chicago. Strictly speaking it is not an arts film, but it carries a profound message about communication and is one of the most enlightened documentaries about dementia yet produced. To see clips from it and/or to purchase go to www. memorybridge.org

There is a DVD of Elderflowers: *Red Nose Coming* available from Dementia Services Development Centre, University of Stirling.

Films

It is also worth having a look at some of the films posted on YouTube. Two short ones about painting which are outstanding and have been professionally made are *Painting in Twilight: An Artist's Escape From Alzheimer's*, and an ABC film from Australia, *Art and Alzheimer's*.

Journals

Journal of Dementia Care is a bi-monthly journal aimed at individuals who work alongside people with dementia. If regularly features and describes a broad range of arts projects undertaken across a range of settings.

Signpost is also an extremely informative journal. Details can be found at www.signpostjournal.org.uk

Useful Websites

There is video material of Ladder to the Moon on their website: www.laddertothemoon.co.uk

www.picturestoshare.co.uk

www.digitaljewellery.com

www.artistsforalzheimers.org [This is an organisation that links artists with people with Alzheimer's disease. The site contains details of work in progress and a wealth of resources and ideas].

www.dementiapositive.co.uk [This is John and Kate Allan's website which is a veritable arts feast with information about inspiring projects and quotes by people with dementia about the arts].

www.timeslips.org [Time Slips is a creative storytelling project. The site contains a wealth of ideas and resources as well as signposts to additional materials].

Social Care Institute for Excellence: Good Practice Example 01 – Improving access to ICT in adult social care setting: www.scie.org. uk/workforce/getconnected/examples/example01 [last accessed 5th February 2011]

www.healthcentral.com

www.heartsminds.org.uk

www.getintoreading.org

www.thrive.org.uk/ Thrive [This organisation provides a range of briefing sheets on the therapeutic use of gardens and gardening.]

www.magicme.co.uk/ [This website shares a range of intergenerational projects.]

www.turtlekeyarts.org.uk

www.morethanmemory.me [This site created by Jayne Wallace and Claire Craig contains a wealth of free, dowloadable materials and ideas.]

Index